THE DYING PROCESS

'I don't like the idea of lingering. If it's going to happen let it happen; not all this hanging on dying inch by inch, fighting every scrap of the way' (hospice patient).

Taking as its focus a highly emotive area of study, *The Dying Process* draws on the experiences of day care and hospice patients to provide a forceful new analysis of the period of decline prior to death.

Placing the bodily realities of dying very firmly centre stage and questioning the ideology central to the modern hospice movement of enabling patients to 'live until they die', Julia Lawton shows how our concept of a 'good death' is open to interpretation. Her study examines the non-negotiable effects of a patient's bodily deterioration on their sense of self and, in so doing, offers a powerful new perspective on embodiment and emotion in death and dying.

A detailed and subtle ethnographic study, *The Dying Process* engages with a range of deeply complex and ethically contentious issues surrounding the care of dying patients in hospices and elsewhere. This book makes a significant contribution to the field of the sociology of the body and will also be an invaluable text for professionals, students and others who wish to enhance their understanding of hospice and palliative care.

Julia Lawton is a Research Fellow at Newnham College, University of Cambridge.

THE DYING PROCESS

Patients' experiences of palliative care

Julia Lawton

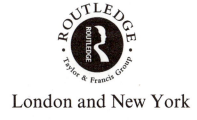

London and New York

First published 2000
by Routledge
11 New Fetter Lane, London EC4P 4EE

Simultaneously published in the USA and Canada
by Routledge
29 West 35th Street, New York, NY 10001

Routledge is an imprint of the Taylor & Francis Group

Typeset in Times by Taylor & Francis Books Ltd
Printed and bound in Great Britain by Clays Ltd, St Ives plc

British Library Cataloguing in Publication Data
A catalogue record for this book is available from the British Library

Library of Congress Cataloging in Publication Data
Lawton, Julia, 1969–
The Dying Process: patients' experiences of palliative care / Julia
Lawton
p. cm.
Includes bibliographical references.
1. Palliative treatment 2. Terminal care. 3. Death. I. Title.
R726.8 L39 2000
362.1'75–dc21
99–087378

ISBN 0–415–22678–3 (hbk)
ISBN 0–415–22679–1 (pbk)

CONTENTS

Preface and acknowledgements   vi

1 Introduction   1

2 Day care: a safe retreat   39

Preface to Chapters 3 and 4 – changing contexts:
entering the hospice   76

3 'Body-subject' to 'body-object': hospice care
and the dying patient   81

4 Inpatient hospice care: the sequestration of the
unbounded body and 'dirty dying'   122

5 Invisible suffering: the social death   148

6 Final reflections   171

Appendix A   187
Appendix B   189
Notes   191
Bibliography   205
Name index   223
Subject index   227

PREFACE AND ACKNOWLEDGEMENTS

Like many people in their twenties, the age I was when I began this study, I had not had any extensive, firsthand exposure to death and dying. True, I lost several elderly relatives during my childhood, but all of these deaths occurred in hospital and none of them seemed very real to me at the time. I did not question why I was not taken to visit my relatives before they died, nor for that matter why I did not attend their funerals; it was just the way things were for children in those days. Apart from these somewhat sheltered experiences, my only other personal encounter with death involved a close friend who died very suddenly and unexpectedly during my first year at university. His death was tragic to say the least, but it was also atypical.

I thus began this study with a certain naïveté, a naïveté which stemmed partly from my personal circumstances, but also from broader social and cultural factors. This naïveté, I hope, has facilitated rather than hindered the observations and arguments developed in this book, for my naïveté (and that of others), as I came realise, was something that required analysis and understanding in its own right.

Like other people in my circumstances, I did not lack a conception of death and dying altogether. Films, TV dramas and novels (even in my early childhood) were filled with images of death: soldiers dying heroically on the battlefields; cowboys and Indians in mortal combat in Westerns; and cops and robbers in armed shootouts. What is notable about these portrayals is that death is seen to occur in an instant, the wounded person staggering slightly before falling to the ground and dying. Running in parallel with these masculine images, more feminised portrayals also occur, such as those contained in Hollywood-style deathbed scenes. In these depictions the heroine (for the dying person in this context is normally a she) is viewed elegantly reclined in bed, hair perfectly in place, surrounded by 'loved ones'. Typically a few tears are shed and farewells said, before our heroine (still looking surprisingly well at the time) rests her head on her pillow, closes her eyes and breathes her last breath. These two seemingly dissimilar portrayals in fact have strong points of affinity: it is not so much what is represented, as what is *not* represented in both, that I came to recognise as significant.

I also read extensively about hospice care before starting the research in earnest. Most of the literature available at that time was written by hospice professionals (a situation which has changed substantially since then), and this literature did little, if anything, to dispel my somewhat untroubled (pre-)conceptions. Here we are told that the dying process that has been hidden away in hospitals is surrounded by problems; problems for which hospice care can provide the solution. The images accessible within this literature are in fact very similar to those contained within Hollywood deathbed scenes. Hospice professionals offer the reassurance that, with the compassionate care and effective methods of pain control they can now provide, it is possible to preserve the dignity of dying patients right up until the point of death; to enable patients to 'live until they die'. A somewhat romanticised conception of dying patients resting comfortably in bed, mentally alert, calm and reassured is all too prevalent within this literature.

I would not say that I bought into the modern hospice movement's vision in its entirety, but I had little, if any, firsthand experience with which to question it. Armed with only the very selective images of death and dying described above, I experienced a real sense of shock once I actually began my fieldwork. I should emphasise right here that I saw nothing but excellent standards of care in the hospice and day care service in which I worked: staff and volunteers in both settings displayed a warmth, humanity and professionalism which I found quite remarkable. What I was unprepared for was somewhat different: it was the visible signs of bodily decay; the stench of incontinence; the lethargy and despondency of patients, many of whom had struggled with their illness for months or years; and the burnout and exhaustion experienced by their families and friends. These realities were often a far cry from the broader stereotypes, for even within the literature written by hospice professionals themselves, the protracted period of suffering that can occur prior to death is rarely, if ever, portrayed. Yet, clearly there are good reasons why such selective and romanticised images exist; there is something very comforting in the belief that the end of life can be a peaceful and dignified affair, that death itself need not be prolonged and unnecessarily drawn out. This, after all, is what we all hope for, not only for ourselves, but also for the people we care about.

Once I had recovered from my initial sense of shock, a new set of problems surfaced. As a participant observer, I spent a great deal of time in close emotional and physical proximity to patients and their families. I grew very fond of some patients and their deaths, though anticipated, were often a source of great sadness and loss. Over 200 patients died during the period of fieldwork, and the accumulative effect of witnessing so many deaths, and the deterioration that often went on beforehand, caused me to feel very despondent by the time I had completed the research.

The difficulties associated with this study have also extended well beyond the fieldwork period. I have, for example, frequently confronted the dilemma of how to present my material and, more importantly, to whom. Presentations of my work have often brought emotional scars to the surface amongst members of the audience, a situation which carries its own responsibilities. It has become an all too common occurrence to be approached by one or more people after a seminar wishing to talk frankly of the anguish they experienced after a family member or friend died in a particularly distressing way. Such encounters point to clear conclusions: whilst the romanticised images of death and dying that are prevalent within society can be helpful and reassuring to many people, they can also lead to false expectations and, ultimately, to a sense of disappointment and disillusionment amongst others. Many of those who approached me felt that they, personally, had failed because their family member or friend had not died in the way that they had expected and hoped for. The reactions of others to my research have been different, but equally strong. For some, the mere mention that I conducted a study in a hospice provokes a terse, 'oh that must be very depressing' and a prompt change of subject. Others still, I know, actively avoid me. The label 'Dr Death', and the stigma associated with it, is one that I have carried with me right from the study's inception.

Not surprisingly then, the research I describe in the following pages was neither easy to carry out nor to write up, and I have many friends and colleagues to thank for both intellectual and emotional support. Two people, in particular, stand out both for their generosity with their time and for the painstaking and extremely helpful comments they have made on early and later versions of this work: Sarah Green and Susan Benson. I consider myself very lucky to have had the opportunity to work with them, both in recent times and at earlier stages in my academic career. Frances Pine, likewise, has been an extremely valued source of support over a period that has now spanned almost ten years. Frances first stimulated my interest in social anthropology, and if it had not been for her academic influence, it is extremely unlikely that this book would ever have been written. I also owe a special debt of gratitude to Marilyn Strathern and Ronnie Frankenberg, both for their incisive and thought provoking comments, and for their more general encouragement and support. Charlotte Carr, too, stands out for particular thanks. She has constantly helped to keep me on my toes, and the dialogue I have had with her has been helpful in developing some of the theoretical ideas contained within this book. Catherine Alexander, Adam Reed and Melissa Nash have also contributed significantly to the final shaping of the manuscript and, as importantly, have been loyal and supportive friends. An additional thank you goes to my anonymous reviewers for their helpful comments.

I have also been extremely lucky to meet a number of helpful and supportive people at forums where earlier versions of this work have been presented. One of the most stimulating venues has been the annual symposium on Social Aspects of Death, Dying and Bereavement, where I have received very helpful feedback on my own material, together with the opportunity to keep up to date with the work of others. I am grateful to all the people I have met at these symposia, but particularly to David Clark, David Field, Jenny Hockey, Jeanne Katz and Tony Walter. Similar support has come from the colleagues I have met through the 'body group' organised by Bryan Turner and Nina Hallowell in Cambridge, together with those based at the Institute of Public Health in Cambridge. I also thank John Goldsmith, Nicky James, Jocalyn Lawler and Frances Price for the good advice they have given me at critical moments.

This study, of course, would not have been possible if it had not been for the kindness and generosity of all those attached to the hospice and day care service in which fieldwork was conducted. Regrettably I cannot thank these particular people by name here, because I have chosen not to disclose the exact location of my fieldwork sites. I will always be particularly indebted to day care's NHS manager, the Senior Consultant in Palliative Medicine, and the head of Research and Development of the local NHS Trust. I cannot thank these three people enough for all the practical help they gave me despite their own hectic work schedules and, more importantly still, for the trust they bestowed in me by allowing the study to proceed. I am also extremely grateful to the staff and volunteers in day care and the hospice, not only for all the insights they shared with me, but also for the kindness they showed me, particularly on occasions when the research caused me to feel very upset. I know there were times when staff found it difficult having a researcher under their feet, but they all showed remarkable patience and good humour, and I consider it a privilege to have been able to work with them.

I am also very grateful to the staff and managers in day care and the hospice for giving me the freedom to develop ideas and to express views, some of which, I know, conflict with their own. I have been given help in clarifying the factual details contained within this book; however, the interpretations and arguments stemming from my observations are entirely my own.

Support of equal importance has also come from other sources. New Hall, Cambridge is remarkable for the generosity it gives to young scholars, and I am very grateful indeed to the college for funding my research. The writing of this book has also been made possible by Newnham College, Cambridge where I currently hold a Research Fellowship, a position which has given me both the time and opportunity to refine my analysis.

My parents and step-parents have been a constant and unerring source of encouragement and support. They know how grateful I am to them. I am also grateful to my friends who have all provided shoulders to lean on, both at times when I found my fieldwork upsetting and on occasions when the writing of this book became very stressful. In addition to those already mentioned, I thank Rachel Austin, Amber Cole, Anya Dathan, Edward Leigh, Alison Meekoff, Claire Somerville, Andrea Stöckl, and Sarah Stringer. A very special thank you goes to William Tunstall-Pedoe for always being there for me, and to my step-father Geoffrey Woodcock for meticulous proof-reading at short notice.

Yet, it is to the patients, their families and friends whose experiences I draw upon in this study that I feel a gratitude that I could not even begin to measure. I cannot thank them enough for their frankness and honesty, and it is to them that I dedicate this book.

Chapter 4 in this book is a revised version of an article originally published as 'Contemporary hospice care: the sequestration of the unbounded body and "dirty dying" ', *Sociology of Health & Illness* 20, 2: 121–43. I am grateful to Blackwell Publishers for allowing me to reproduce this material.

1

INTRODUCTION

Introductory remarks

This book aims to substantially revise concepts of the 'Western' self through an analysis of empirical research on the experiences of dying patients receiving palliative care in contemporary England. There is now a proliferation of sociological and cultural studies on the 'Western' self and its relationship to the body (e.g. Giddens 1991; Falk 1994; Featherstone *et al.* 1993; Shilling 1993; Turner 1984), yet few of these explore the process by which people negotiate and understand themselves in practice in their daily lives, let alone during traumatic moments such as the period of decline and deterioration leading towards death. Through closely detailed ethnographic research, this study both contextualises these intellectual debates and challenges some of their underlying presuppositions. In particular, it focuses on concepts of the person, and the importance of certain physical capacities and boundaries for the maintenance of the 'Western' self. As the research described in this book reveals, many characteristics central to the 'Western' self only become visible after they have been lost, as it were. It is for this reason that a study of dying patients has a unique and important contribution to make to these debates.

Whilst particular attention is focused upon the ways in which patients' experiences of self, body, space and time shift and change during the period between receiving a diagnosis of terminal disease and their eventual bed-ridden deaths, the study also highlights and explores several other related themes. One of these, rarely analysed, is the question of the 'intersubjectivity' and 'intercorporeality' of the process of dying. To look at this, the study sets patients' experiences alongside those of family and friends, allowing an

1

analysis of the complex ways in which patients' deterioration affects the bodies, selves and identities of those involved with their care. This aspect of the study draws out the importance of intersubjective and intercorporeal experiences, and, in so doing, destabilises the notion that the 'Western' self is always and necessarily coherent, unified and self-contained within the parameters of a single body.

Moreover, the research outlined in the pages that follow highlights the difficulties of matching the modern hospice movement's ideological goal of enabling patients to 'live until they die' with the realities of the ways in which many patients cared for in hospices bodily degenerate ('rot away and die') in practice. This disparity between the rhetorics and the realities of hospice care is not only noted through ethnographic description; it is also analysed through the context in which it occurs.

Detailed descriptions are provided of patients' experiences at various stages in their illness and deterioration, thereby bringing the human reality of these events to the fore in the text. By combining these descriptions with broader theoretical perspectives, this study aims to give the reader both an empathetic and analytical understanding of the perspectives of 'the dying' and those involved with their care. One of the central and fundamentally important arguments of the book which arises from this approach is that during the course of their illness and bodily deterioration, patients may lose various aspects of their selfhood and identity which qualify them for the status of a 'person'.[1] In other words, it is possible for a patient to die socially – that is, to enter the realms of non-personhood – prior to his or her physical cessation.[2] By identifying those capacities and attributes which, when lost, erode a patient's ability to be themselves and to be seen as such by others, this study provides far reaching insights into what in fact makes a person a *person* within modern 'Western' contexts.

The focus on the centrality of the body, as a physical entity, to contemporary concepts of person and self is a key aspect to the research, and this focus, as we shall see, transcends existing literature on embodiment in a number of ways. For example, by making the 'non-negotiable', deteriorating bodies of dying patients a central point of analysis, this study provides a critique of the ways in which post-modern thinkers have tended to theorise the self as operating through the construction and presentation of a 'performative' body. Such a theorisation, it will be shown, is often not a demonstration of the inadequacy of mind–body dualism as these authors intended, but is instead a reiteration of that very dualism. Aspects of embodiment hitherto kept in the background, such as the capacity for mobility and for corporeal 'self-containment', are revealed through this research to be absolutely fundamental to selfhood in modern 'Western' contexts. The book thus argues that a fundamental rethinking of the intellectual understanding of the relationship between the body and the self is needed.

The research begins in a day care service for patients who had received a recent diagnosis of incurable disease, and whose illness had begun to undermine their capacity to function normally. The study then moves into an inpatient hospice which caters for patients during the last stages of their illness, and was the place in which many patients finally died. Consideration is paid to the various ways in which medical advances, changing funding strategies within the NHS, and other social and political forces affected the difficult and complex decisions which surrounded the treatment and management of patients in both settings. In so doing, this study directly engages with a range of complex and ethically contentious debates which centre upon the care of dying patients in hospices and other locations.

Whilst this study was conducted in one regional location, contemporary England, it is hoped that the observations and analyses developed will have broader applications, contributing, for example, to debates on the 'Western' self in the ways indicated above. It is important to recognise, however, that terms such as 'the West' and 'the Western person' are inherently problematic, because anthropologists (and others) who have used – and continue to use – these stereotypes often appear to assume that 'the West' is an homogenous area characterised by uniform features (see Moore 1994: 131). Whilst the 'West' is thus perhaps more an intellectual construction than an empirical reality, such a concept will be used (with caution) in the pages that follow.[3]

This introductory chapter provides the necessary background for the book as a whole, and sets the context for the chapters which follow. In it, I provide an analysis of how the 'management' of death and dying has changed during this century, and point to the various social and cultural forces which supposedly stimulated the development of the modern hospice movement in the UK. The day care and inpatient services where I conducted fieldwork are then located, described and examined within the broader context of the hospice movement, its ideology and philosophy of care, and its development over time. This examination is followed by a description of the methods I used to collect data within day care and the hospice, together with some reflections upon the 'typicality' of the patients to whom I had access during the period of field-work. The chapter concludes by outlining the following chapters, and highlights the ways in which they relate to and connect with one another. I begin by considering the concepts of 'person', 'self' and 'identity', as they are used, understood and critiqued within this study.

Person, self and identity

Whilst there has been broad agreement amongst anthropologists that what constitutes and characterises 'human beings' is subject to cultural and historical variability (see, for example, Mauss 1985; Dumont 1985) the actual terminology used to describe and understand these 'human beings', as La Fontaine (1985: 124) points out, has been a matter of some confusion and debate. In light of such confusion, La Fontaine suggests that it is most fruitful to draw a distinction between what she terms the 'individual', defined as, 'the mortal human being, the object of observation' (1985: 126) on the one hand, and the 'person' on the other, the latter term being used 'to refer to concepts ... which lend the object social significance' (ibid.).[4] Such a distinction is useful because it allows for the idea that one can be a 'mortal human being' without necessarily being a person, since entry into personhood requires certain culturally dictated criteria to be possessed and/or achieved. Certainly, Fortes, in his study of the Tallensi of Ghana, has argued that marriage and the birth of children were essential prerequisites for a member of that society to attain personhood, the implication being that not all members of the Tallensi were persons (Fortes 1973). In a similar manner, the observations and analyses developed within this book will suggest that in contexts such as contemporary England, adults can continue to exist as living human beings *after* they have lost those bodily and social attributes which allow them to be seen, and to see themselves, as persons.

Yet the separation between the 'individual', 'the object of observation' and the person has itself recently come under attack in the work of academics such as Strathern (1988). Such a distinction, Strathern argues, is inherently problematic because it contains within it the assumption that the person is always and necessarily a distinct, integrated, unified whole, contained within a singular

4

body; a unified entity, furthermore, which can be set against a wider social whole, 'as in our contrasting ideas about society working upon individuals and individuals shaping society' (1988: 13). This conception, she suggests, is ethnocentric, stemming from 'Western' stereotypical understandings of the person, and thus cannot be assumed to exist cross-culturally; an observation which has also been echoed by Shore (1982: 133). Whilst the cross-cultural existence of the 'individual' has now been subjected to extensive critical scrutiny (see Chapter 3), this study will explore the extent to which the stereotype does, or does not, actually conform to practices and self-understandings amongst 'Western' persons themselves. Because we will in fact see instances wherein selfhood appears to be experienced in fluid, overlapping ways which extend beyond the parameters of an 'individuated' body, the term 'individual' will not be used extensively and unreflexively within this study.

The person of modern 'Western' contexts, as various academics have argued, is composed of two separate but interdependent components: an identity and a self (see, for example, Giddens 1991; Rose 1990; Morris 1994: 14). The self is one's inner subjective being; it is an essence which, in this particular cultural and historical context, is interior to the subject/person (Taylor 1985). Identity, on the other hand is externally dictated; it is derived from the cultural meanings and community memberships that others confer upon a societal member. In other words, identities develop both in stable roles and in the emergent situations of social interaction (Goffman 1959); identity is what is draped over participants by the social and cultural group they are in, and varies according to one's context at any given time (see, for example, Lloyd 1993; Jackson 1996: 26). In practice, however, one's self and one's identity are often fundamentally entwined since, just as the 'presentation of self' (Goffman 1959) involves the negotiation and projection of one's inner sense to the outside world and thus constitutes a part of one's identity,[5] one's identity or identities can become, to some extent, internalised and thus part of one's self-concept (Mead 1934). Certainly, as later observations and analyses will suggest, whilst members of contemporary 'Western' societies often conceive of themselves as unique and autonomous entities, such a notion of person and self is often dependent upon, and realised through, interpersonal relationships which are themselves based upon a certain level of mutual autonomy.[6] Consequently, the modern 'Western' self, in the sense used in this study, involves a blending of interior and exterior (relational) components, and without these components there can be no person.

Whilst there is a substantial and internally highly varied literature outside social anthropology which traces the emergence of the modern sense of 'Western' personhood (see, for example, Taylor 1989; Elias 1994; Foucault 1987; Rose 1990, 1996; Lukes 1973), within the discipline itself greatest attention to this phenomenon has been paid by writers such as Mauss (1985) and Dumont (1985). Both have, in similar ways, pointed to broader cultural changes and, in particular, to the transition they see as having occurred from 'holistic' societies based on ascribed statuses to 'individualistic', achievement-based societies. With such a transition, they argue, modern 'Western' persons have ceased to be enmeshed within kinship structures and other political, economic and religious systems which define and constrain who and what they are: as Dumont suggests, the 'individual' him or herself, rather than 'society', has now become the 'paramount value' (1985: 94; see also Macfarlane 1978). With this loosening of the external moral grip of society, as both academics further observe, the person not only begins to emerge as a differentiated 'individual', he or she also becomes endowed with a moral value and a moral consciousness, with 'individual rights' and 'self-interests', that are separate from any social roles that are occupied (see also Lukes 1985; Morris 1994: 153). Person and self, in other words, become merged in distinctive ways, a phenomenon which explains why the two concepts can, and often are, used interchangeably in the modern 'West'.[7] Indeed, as Mauss notes: 'the "person" (*personne*) [now] equals the "self" (*moi*); the "self" (*moi*) equals consciousness, and is its primordial category' (1985: 21, original emphasis). Such a conception of the 'Western' person/self, as Rose's study neatly sums up, is one which is perceived in academic discourse as being 'coherent, bounded, individualised, intentional, the locus of thought, action and belief, the origin of its own actions, the beneficiary of a unique biography' (1996: 3).

Yet, as I indicated above, one of the objectives of this book is to use the observations and analyses developed to address broader intellectual concerns, in particular to provide a critique of the ways in which concepts of the 'Western' person/self have been used and theorised within the academic literature. At a time when anthropologists are more frequently applying their ethnographic skills 'at home' (for example, Strathern 1992a, 1992b; La Fontaine 1996; Franklin 1997), their observations are beginning to reveal a much more complex picture of 'Western' personhood than has hitherto been assumed. Indeed, Bloch has recently observed that, 'the individualism of the west needs to be greatly qualified. It is more self description than a sociological finding and the fragility of its ideology emerges at every turn' (1988: 28).

The distinction drawn between 'self description' and 'sociological (read: empirical) finding' is a crucial one because it highlights the problems of assuming that the theoretical models of the 'Western' person/self derived from 'serious discourse' (B. Morris 1991: 271) and enshrined in legislation (Moore 1994: 35) are an accurate reflection of the everyday experiences and practices. By exploring the ways in which selfhood is lived *and lost* in practice in contemporary England, this study reveals a somewhat complex and internally varied picture: a picture which suggests that no simple distinction can be drawn between 'high theory' on the one hand and 'folk' understandings on the other.[8] On the contrary, it appears that the ways in which ordinary people in England perceive and evaluate themselves and others are shaped by a conceptual framework which is composed of certain strands of both (see Moore 1994: 35). Consequently, whilst there are some contexts in which contemporary English conceptions of person and self seem to conform to what Battaglia has termed a 'rhetorics of individuality' (1995: 3), in other contexts such a stereotype will be shown to be problematic.

One of the central problems with most theoretical models, as this study will highlight, is that they are premised upon an essentially 'disembodied' conception of the person/self. What remains implicit in such models – but will be made absolutely explicit in this work – is that in order for selfhood to be realised and maintained in contexts such as contemporary England, certain specific bodily capacities and attributes *must* be possessed: the most important being a bounded, physically sealed, enclosed body (what I term the corporeal capacity for 'self-containment'), and also the bodily ability to act as the agent of one's embodied actions and intentions. Patients[9] who lose either, or both of these bodily attributes, as we shall see, fall out of the category of personhood in both their own and other people's evaluations; they experience a diminishment of self. It will thus be one of the aims of this book to revise and extend existing theoretical paradigms to incorporate more of a 'bodily element'. In so doing, this study will also provide a powerful critique of recent sociological work on the body (e.g. Featherstone *et al.* 1993; Falk 1994; Shilling 1993). Whilst the authors of these studies have also attempted to make the body of the modern 'Western' person visible, the emphasis given in their work to the 'performative' aspects of embodiment presents, as indicated above, a somewhat partial picture.

Yet it is not enough to bring the body fully into frameworks of observation and analysis: as the experiences of the patients described in this book will also be used to highlight, bodies, in practice, cannot usually be considered in isolation from interpersonal relationships, since both, in interdependent ways, are central to contemporary 'Western' formations and conceptions of self. By making the connections between bodies and relationships explicit, this work constitutes a significant theoretical advance on social studies of embodiment, and on those studies which explore the role of intimacy and emotions in the making of self through social interconnection (e.g. Giddens 1991, 1993).

I now turn to the development of the modern hospice movement, since both the day care service and inpatient facility where I conducted research were located under the umbrella of this particular organisation. The modern hospice movement afforded a particularly appropriate context within which to pursue the theoretical objectives of this book since, as we shall see, there is embedded within the hospice philosophy of care a similar 'rhetorics of individuality' to that contained within the academic models outlined above. In practice, this meant that staff in both the hospice and the day care service confronted substantial difficulties aligning the formal goals and objectives of the modern hospice movement with the realities of how personhood is actually lived – and lost – in the modern English setting; difficulties which will be highlighted and analysed in later chapters.

The shifting context of death and dying during the twentieth century

In order to understand the goals and objectives of the modern hospice movement it is necessary to locate them within the context of the various socio-historical forces which stimulated the movement's development. According to the historical record, a significant transition has occurred during the past fifty or so years in the ways in which death and dying have been located, handled and managed within 'Western' contexts.[10] As Ariès (1981) observes, from the fifth to the nineteenth century in European civilisation, death was confronted on an open and regular basis because people normally died in their own homes, surrounded by members of their family and community. It was also common practice for the body of the deceased to be 'laid-out' at home, after which visits were made by family, friends and others to view and touch the corpse (Cline 1995: 43). Death and dying, as a consequence, were seen as a normal and natural part of life; an integral part of everyday existence (Ariès 1981; see also Kearl 1989; Richardson 1989). The twentieth century, however, has seen the emergence of the supposedly 'hidden death' (Ariès 1981: 570), a phenomenon which occurs within a medical setting and which 'began very discreetly in the 1930s and 40s and became widespread after 1950' (ibid.). As Field and James note, by the mid-1960s two-thirds of all deaths in the UK occurred in hospitals and other places caring for the sick (e.g. nursing homes); a figure which had risen to 71 per cent by 1989 (1993: 8). In this way, home, 'the space in which living takes place' (Hockey 1990: 36), has become 'inappropriate as a space for dying' (ibid.).

A number of factors have been highlighted which are believed to have encouraged the removal of death and dying from the home to the hospital. It has been suggested, for example, that the processes of secularisation have resulted in a transition from a religious to a medical framework in the management of death (Hockey 1990: 56), with the doctor, rather than the priest, overseeing the dying process (Walter 1994: 12).[11] In a more practical sense, developments in medical, surgical and pharmacological technology have stimulated the move to hospital-based deaths, because it is within medical institutions that most medical equipment and expertise are concentrated (Field and James 1993: 12; Ariès 1981: 584; see also Foucault 1993). Field and James also point to changing family and occupational structures as being key to this process (1993: 6). As they suggest, smaller families and the fragmentation of the family unit due to the increased social and geographical mobility of its members, coupled with the increased involvement of women in the labour market, have had the effect of causing 'a progressive reduction in the availability of unpaid lay carers' able to look after a dying patient at home (1993: 7). Indeed, as Neale observes, the admission of a dying person to a medical or residential unit may have more to do with the inability of family members to care for him or her at home than it does with the needs and condition of the patient *per se* (1993: 53). Such a problem, as Seale further points out, has been compounded by a rise in the average life expectancy of the population, which has led to an increasing proportion of chronically ill elderly people requiring time consuming care (1990).

The removal of death and dying from the home to medical institutions has resulted not only in a spatial, but also in a reconfigured symbolic separation between life and death (Hockey 1990: 36). As Backer observes, the institutionalisation of death and dying has resulted in these processes becoming largely invisible to most people within society (1982: 10). Consequently, at the same time as death and dying were removed from mainstream social life, a silence developed around these topics: as Ariès suggests, the sequestration of death has led to it replacing sex as the main cultural taboo within the 'West' (Ariès 1981; see also Gorer 1965). Such an observation helps to explain why, by the 1960s, it had become extremely rare to inform dying patients of their prognosis (Glaser and Strauss 1966: 5). Patients were kept in ignorance of their impending deaths, partly to spare their own feelings, but also so that their family and doctors could avoid discussing a subject which they now found very discomforting (Ariès 1981: 561).

The 'hospitalisation of death', however, brought about a somewhat paradoxical situation since medical institutions were not actually geared in cultural or personal terms to the care of dying patients. As Hockey argues: 'Given that traditional medical models are either preventative or curative, neither therefore addresses themselves directly to managing the implacable and incurable processes of dying and bereavement' (1990: 63). Within a medical framework, death was thus seen as failure by practitioners (Backer 1982: 10). It is perhaps not surprising, therefore, that the small number of sociological studies which looked at the care of dying patients in hospitals during the 1960s revealed the somewhat 'inhuman' ways in which patients were 'managed' by medical staff (see, for example, Glaser and Strauss 1966; Sudnow 1967). These studies indicated that a hospital's technical orientation to patient care both alienated the dying patient and facilitated his or her sense of personal isolation and powerlessness. Not only did medical professionals rarely inform dying patients of their prognosis, they often avoided contact with such patients altogether (Glaser and Strauss 1965: 5). It was also common practice to sedate patients very heavily, partly because medical staff had no adequate means of controlling their physical pain, but also to reduce the likelihood that patients would read the 'fateful signs' of impending death (Glaser and Strauss 1966: 40). Sudnow's observational study of American hospitals showed that once a patient had been sedated into a pre-comatose state, from then on staff often regarded him or her as a corpse. It was not uncommon, for example, for staff to close a patient's eyes prior to death, since this was a much more difficult task to perform once that patient had died (1967: 74). Yet, as Walter argues, most studies of the changing management of death and dying should be treated with some degree of scepticism, because there would seem to be embedded within them a certain sense of nostalgia, a 'harking back to a pre-modern era, before the scientific and medical discourses of modernity "ruined" dying' (1993: 286). A similar opinion is expressed by Elias who focuses his critical attention upon Ariès' historical studies. 'Ariès' selection of facts', he suggests, 'is based upon a preconceived opinion. ... In a Romantic spirit Ariès looks mistrustfully on the bad present in the name of a better past' (1985: 12). Such a phenomenon, as we shall see below, does not appear to be confined solely within the academic literature: hospice proponents, in their writings, also seem to have represented the past in a somewhat selective manner. It may well be the case that the pioneers of the movement have also, to an extent, 'invented tradition' (Hobsbawm and Ranger 1983); editing and reconstructing the past or pasts in such a way as to bolster and legitimate the contemporary goals of modern hospice care.

The development of the modern hospice movement in the UK

The modern hospice movement developed in the late 1960s in the UK, stimulated in the first instance by a small number of medical professionals who had themselves become very disillusioned with the care of dying patients in hospitals. Like the academic researchers referred to above, hospice pioneers pointed to severe shortcomings in the ways in which dying patients were cared for at the time by medical staff. One of their common complaints, for example, was that dying patients were moved to remote corners of wards or into side rooms, with visits from medical staff becoming progressively 'cursory' and 'infrequent' (Twycross 1992: 5). Similarly, because a patient was rarely informed of his or her prognosis: 'The patient feels he [sic] doesn't matter anymore. Although it is his illness, he is not consulted about anything, his co-operation is not sought' (ibid.). Hospice proponents also expressed extreme concern about inadequate pain control. They complained that patients were either left alone, terrified, and in a constant state of pain, or they were kept heavily drugged, which meant they remained unconscious or semi-unconscious until they finally died (see du Boulay 1985: 1).

The initial impetus for the modern hospice movement was provided by Cicely Saunders, who was responsible for the founding of St Christopher's hospice in London in 1967. St Christopher's hospice, as I discuss below, quickly became a model or prototype for future developments, inspiring other groups of people across the country to set up their own services (Lunt 1985: 753). The movement provided a radical critique of the supposedly imper-sonal, medicalised, technological management of death occurring within hospitals (James 1994: 103; Abel 1986: 71; Moller 1996: 39). Instead of regarding death as failure, as many hospital doctors appeared to do, hospice pioneers argued that death should be regarded as a normal and natural part of life (Twycross 1992: 6). Consequently, hospice philosophy gave emphasis to care rather than cure, and to the quality rather than the quantity of a patient's life: patients were neither subjected to aggressive life-sustaining strategies nor to excessive technological interventions during the final weeks or days of life (Munley 1983: 35; DuBois 1980: 73–4).

Hospice advocates sought to provide patients with a more personal form of care by stressing the importance of including the family as well as the dying person in the main unit of care (DuBois 1980: 12). This objective was combined with the idea that the hospice staff should provide an environment which, as far as possible, mimicked that of an extended family (Munley 1983: 95). Indeed, it was Saunders' explicit intention that St Christopher's hospice should grow into a 'real community', becoming 'the kind of family and home that can give the kind of welcome and hospitality of a good home' (Saunders 1965). In this respect at least, the modern hospice movement has been interpreted as 'anti-modernist' because of the emphasis it gives to supposedly traditional values such as family networks, community affiliation and a community's responsibility for offering support to those such as the dying and the bereaved (James 1994: 107; Walter 1993: 286; 1994: 42; Owens 1995: 180). As Munley suggests: 'Hospice strikes a responsive chord in people who lament the gradual erosion of many modes of support once provided by family and community' (1983: 95).

Yet in other respects, the emergence of the modern hospice movement can be understood as a direct and explicit response to the development of the modern conception of the self, rather than being simply a reaction to the limitations of hospital culture *per se* (see Walter 1994: 42). Hospice pioneers advocated a model of care in which patients were informed frankly and openly of their condition, and were actively encouraged to participate in all the decisions surrounding their treatment and care (Abel 1986: 73). Hence, one sees a distinct congruence here between the hospice concept and the contemporary notion of the consuming and choosing self as discussed by writers such as Rose (1990; 1996) and Giddens (1991). Indeed, one of the central goals of the modern hospice movement, as Kearl highlights, is to enable patients to retain control of their lives until death (1989: 439), since their 'basic human rights are seen to be violated when they lack the knowledge and power to make decisions' (1989: 438).[12] The hospice movement, in the same spirit, pioneered more effective forms of pain control as an additional way of helping dying patients to retain a sense of control. Hospice doctors devised new methods of administering narcotics and analgesics which made it possible for patients to be kept free of pain, but to still remain lucid and alert (Saunders 1986: 29). 'Freedom from pain while in a conscious and alert state', as Skinner Cook and Oltjenburns suggest, 'allows dying patients to retain control over as much of their lives as possible and to complete their unfinished business prior to death' (1989: 6). Yet if 'retaining control' was one aspect of personhood striven for in a patient's approach to death, it was also assumed that the patient would want to engage in meaningful relationships with others (see above).

Another way in which hospice care sought to 'humanise' the dying process was through the concept of 'total pain'. Hospice proponents criticised hospital practitioners for focusing exclusively upon the treatment and control of a patient's disease; in other words, for treating a patient as a bundle of physical symptoms, rather than as a 'whole person' with a complex and interdependent array of social and emotional needs (see Field and James 1993: 12). In opposition to this conception, hospice pioneers developed and adhered to the Gestaltian notion that a dying patient's physical, emotional, social and spiritual concerns were inextricably entwined, each contributing to their 'total pain experience'; a perspective which confounds the conventional medical model, as well as broader Cartesian notions of a mind–body dualism (Saunders 1993a; O'Brien 1993). In practice, hospice proponents sought to provide 'whole person' care by developing a multi-disciplinary approach, with teams consisting not only of doctors and nurses, but also of other professionals such as chaplains, social workers, counsellors, physiotherapists and occupational therapists, who worked jointly with patients and their families on a non-hierarchical basis (Mulkay 1993: 200–1). Such an approach sought to reintegrate the patient's mind, bodily and spiritual experiences, whilst simultaneously according patients central control over how their care was orchestrated.

When one examines other alternative institutions and reform movements which were beginning to rise into prominence in the 1960s and 1970s, it becomes evident that modern hospices formed part of a broader cluster of social movements which shared a number of features in common (Abel 1986: 71). There is, for example, a distinct parallel between the hospice and the alternative health movement, since both advocate that patients should be viewed as 'whole' human beings (Coward 1989: 44), and that the hierarchical relationship between the 'professional' and the 'patient' should be broken down (Sharma 1992: 203). The women's health movement also challenged the sovereignty of physicians and the technological focus of modern medicine (Abel 1986: 81), with the natural childbirth movement in particular emphasising a woman's right to be fully informed, fully conscious and to experience childbirth as a 'natural' rather than a technological process (Treichler 1990: 121; Coward 1989: 155). All these movements combine anti-modernist strands with a thoroughly modern view of the self both as an author of acts and as a 'consumer' with 'rights'.[13]

In light of the above discussion, the modern hospice movement could be understood as an 'anti-institution', designed to develop rather than to mortify the self of the dying patient (Walter 1994: 54). Indeed, the following 'pledge' offered by the movement's founder Cicely Saunders makes such a goal explicit:

> You matter because you are you.
> You matter to the last moment of your life,
> and we will do all we can
> not only to help you die peacefully,
> but to *live until you die.*
>
> (Saunders, cited in Twycross (1986: 19); emphasis added)

The provision of hospice care, as its proponents further suggested, could enable dying to become a period of 'growth and reconciliation' (Murphy 1993: 131), 'the chance of a creative moment' (Saunders 1988);[14] the implication being that the re-empowerment of dying patients involves a concept of self which is both autonomous and embedded within relationships.

A second radical strand of hospice philosophy centred upon the idea that hospices should manage death in an open rather than a covert fashion.[15] The pioneers of the movement argued that many people had come to fear death because the hospitalisation of dying patients had made it into an invisible, and thus an unknown, entity: as Twycross, a follower of Saunders, suggested:

> half a century ago ... Adults and children alike rubbed shoulders with death and, in so doing, kept the natural fear of death within bounds. Now, for many, divorce from death has resulted in an exaggerated fear coupled with unfamiliarity, awkwardness and embarrassment.
>
> (Twycross 1986: 5)

Hospice professionals, by contrast, advocated an 'open confrontation with death' (Seale 1989: 552). Their rationale was very simple: by breaking the taboo which surrounded death it would be possible to 'expose it as something which is not to be feared and which can be talked about' (Honeybun et al. 1992: 67). Thus proponents emphasised the benefits that patients and others could gain by witnessing another patient die peacefully beside them (Smith 1989: 151; Twycross 1992: 16; Kastenbaum and Aisenberg 1974: 480). This aspect of hospice philosophy was also rooted in Christian beliefs: beliefs which were openly acknowledged by both the founder Cicely Saunders and her followers (Saunders 1965, 1986; Twycross 1986: 28). According to a Christian perspective, death is seen as 'an event in life; not a terminus' (Twycross 1992: 6; see also Smith 1989: 3; Saunders 1988). Hence, as Hockey observes, the hospice movement sought 'to reintegrate the two categories of experience, "life" and "death", thereby highlighting the processual rather than the oppositional nature of their relationship' (1990: 155).

These intertwining beliefs and philosophies have been fed into the 'material ideology' (Miller 1988) of hospice buildings and the working practices taking place within them. Hospices have been designed to house the majority of their patients in communal wards, typically containing anything from three to six beds.[16] Coupled with this design, hospices have a working policy of keeping patients in wards when their conditions become terminal, rather than moving them into side rooms to die (Fagerhaugh and Strauss 1977: 169). Consequently, in the hospice observed during my fieldwork, as in other hospices, there was no overt policy of placing terminal patients in side rooms and, typically, several deaths would occur in the wards each week. Often the curtains around the patient's beds were kept open throughout the time he or she was dying, so that the patient was fully visible to other patients and visitors present in the ward.

The ethics and impact of keeping dying patients on wards will be examined in Chapter 3 where I question whether this is in fact an aspect of hospice ideology which negates, rather than develops, the self of the patient concerned. Indeed, as later chapters make apparent, the central core of this book could be read as a critique of the hospice goal of enabling patients to 'live until they die': a critique which stems in part from my earlier observation that the movement's goals are premised upon somewhat problematic 'rhetorics of individuality', which rest upon a 'disembodied' conception of the person. Certainly, whilst 'death is almost defined as a psychological rather than a physical process' within many hospice formulations (Walter 1994: 30), my fieldwork observations will highlight the absolutely fundamental, non-negotiable undermining impact a patient's bodily deterioration can have upon his or her self. What seems to be 'glossed over' or ignored within the hospice model, then, is the bodily realities of a patient's deterioration and decline: realities which, as we shall see, make it very difficult to enact the goals of hospice care *in practice*. Further difficulties, as I also examine, stem from the wider cultural context within which the movement is located. Whilst proponents also sought to re-empower the dying patient by providing him or her with a 'temporary surrogate family', such a goal is, in reality, confounded by the constant economic pressures placed upon staff to discharge patients. Such pressures, as we shall see, have been exacerbated by recent cutbacks and reforms within the NHS, which severely curtail the *choices* patients are able to exercise over where they are cared for during their last months, weeks and days of life.

Many members of the general population, as I highlight further below, have 'bought into' the hospice vision that 'death can be transformed into a final frontier of self-expression and self-exposition' (Moller 1996: 58). Yet it will be one of my contentions in this book that the widespread popularity behind the modern hospice movement stems partly from the fact that it has propagated an image of death that most people now want to 'consume'; an image which is, in some respects, compatible with contemporary ideas of personhood.

The expansion and transformation of the modern hospice movement in the UK

Like the other alternative institutions and reform movements described above, the hospice movement received widespread popular support at a 'grass roots' level; support which explains the vigorous growth and diversification of the movement's provision since the late 1960s. As James describes, over the past few decades, 'energetic community groups – schools, churches, women's groups, rotarians – have joined with major charities, NHS staff and eventually government to plan and finance a thirty-fold increase in hospice provision' (1994: 102). From their inception, most hospices were dependent not only upon voluntary contributions to provide initial capital and running costs, they also relied strongly upon unpaid volunteers to perform a wide variety of tasks such as counselling patients, transporting patients to and from the hospice and staffing reception points (Field and Johnson 1993: 198, 200). The ideas of the hospice movement, then, were clearly ideas that many ordinary people identified with.

Indeed, in spite of the period of economic depression that occurred during the early 1970s, a large number of local groups and charitable organisations successfully raised the money necessary 'to build a hospice'. Yet, because most of these initiatives were brought about by individuals and groups at a local level, the rapidly expanding movement lacked an overarching organisational framework. Local groups often had little idea how their hospice provision would fit in with other kinds of service both locally and elsewhere (Lunt 1985: 754). Further problems stemmed from the fact that, while it was relatively easy to raise the money necessary to establish new hospice facilities, many schemes were beginning to run up ever larger deficits to meet running costs (Taylor 1983: 17). Consequently, the NHS was being placed under increasing pressure to maintain services which it had neither initially planned nor established: by the 1980s virtually all hospices came to rely upon the NHS for at least partial assistance with their running costs.

It was largely due to these organisational and economic pressures that, from the mid- to late 1970s, the content and structure of the hospice movement began to change quite rapidly. One of the most substantial changes involved the progressive incorporation of hospice units into the economic and organisational framework of the NHS. Lack of co-ordination and disparity in service provision prompted the decision of one of the main charitable organisations, the National Society for Cancer Relief (NSCR), to provide the capital for hospice services only if they were built within the grounds of NHS hospitals, and on the understanding that the health authorities would take responsibility for the full running costs. 'This policy', as Taylor suggests, in part 'indicates the desire of NSCR to influence practice within the NHS, but also reflects a realistic appreciation of the need to secure running costs in the future' (1983: 40). The first NHS hospice was founded in 1975, and by the time I began my fieldwork in 1994, fifty out of the total of 193 inpatient hospice services received joint or separate funding from the NHS and NSCR.[17]

The reforms that have taken place within the NHS since 1991 have brought palliative care services ever further into its organisational framework (I should add here that 'hospice care' and 'palliative care' are now commonly thought to be synonymous, although palliative medicine in fact only became an accredited medical speciality in 1987 (Ahmedzai 1993; Clark and Seymour 1999)). The NHS now works on a contract basis with a variety of service 'providers' competing in the market place for funding from NHS 'purchasing' bodies (Clark 1993: 174).[18] In order to secure either full or partial funding from the NHS, all hospices, including those in the independent sector, must sign a contract with a health authority or other 'purchaser', committing them to provide care of a certain type, standard and cost, and to demonstrate that the standards are being achieved by means of an audit or evaluation (Walter 1994: 167; Neale 1993: 60).

Since the late 1970s and early 1980s, there has also been a diversification of hospice provision, with a shift in emphasis away from the establishment and funding of inpatient units to the provision of home care, day care and other services (Griffin 1991; Seale 1989). Lunt explains this shift as stemming in part from the fact that, by the 1980s, central government policy on health service funding has limited the ability of health authorities to commit themselves to paying the revenue costs of inpatient units (1985: 755). Taylor similarly suggests that the emphasis the hospice movement now places on home care and day care 'follows in the footsteps of similar developments in the NHS towards early discharge of patients into the community ... in order to release expensive in-patient beds and maintain patients where they prefer to be – in their own homes' (1983: 32).[19] Consequently, it has increasingly become the normal practice of general practitioners to keep patients at home for as long as possible, and only to admit them to inpatient units for short periods and during the final and most distressing stages of their illness (Taylor 1983: 15).

A number of hospice professionals and researchers have expressed concern about the impact these economic and organisational changes have had upon the hospice movement (Clark 1993; Wilkes 1993). Because the movement started off as a critique of the practices occurring within hospitals, it initially, and intentionally, developed outside the framework of the NHS.[20] However, as we have seen, hospice services are progressively 'entering into partnership with the same system that they broke away from' (Ahmedzai 1993: 142); a partnership which, as some writers have suggested, may cause their overriding ideological goals to become compromised. James, for example, has pointed to the 'routinisation' that can occur within NHS-sponsored hospices, with a shift in emphasis taking place from the spiritual, emotional and social care of dying patients to a concentration upon their physical symptoms (James 1986, 1994; see also Johnson *et al.* 1990; Wilkes 1993: 2; Abel 1986). Neale has expressed similar concern about the impact of current auditing procedures which, she suggests, 'may not be sensitive enough to measure the intangible, informal qualities of care so valued in early hospices' (1993: 60). As Walter has likewise argued, 'it is easier to demonstrate effective pain control, high bed occupancy and financial cost per patient than to demonstrate real attentiveness to patients' wishes' (1994: 167).[21] The difficulties with which the movement now has to contend have been theorised by some writers through the use of fairly unreflexive gender stereotypes. It has been suggested, for instance, that hospice care developed as an essentially 'feminine' (Walter 1994: 169) and 'maternal' (Moller 1996: 60) response to the 'depersonalisation of male technological rationality' (Walter 1994: 71). Consequently, various problems are arising now that hospice services are being progressively drawn back into a 'masculine' framework; in this case, a framework characterised by the concerns of cost-effectiveness and cost-accountability (Hugman 1994).

The tensions occurring within the UK hospice movement can be found elsewhere: Torrens, for example, in his overview of the hospice movement in America, has argued that modern hospices now rest uncomfortably between 'two worlds' and two opposing views of 'reality' – what he terms the 'emotional' and the 'economic' (1986: 6). Such diametrically opposed 'realities', as he further suggests, 'often pull hospice workers in entirely different directions' (ibid.). Nevertheless, the specific nature of the UK situation must be emphasised here; in particular, the relationship that now exists between the modern hospice movement and the NHS. As later chapters illustrate, an underlying and often irreconcilable conflict did appear to exist between the staff and the NHS management in both the day care service and the inpatient hospice where I conducted fieldwork. Whilst staff were anxious to provide their patients with 'a safe haven' and a 'surrogate family', their goals came into constant conflict with the managerial objective of 'processing patient case loads' as 'efficiently' and 'cost-effectively' as possible.[22] Such a conflict is one of the recurrent themes that runs through the pages that follow.

Setting the fieldwork sites in context

The hospice

The hospice where I conducted fieldwork was first opened in 1981, at a time when the hospice movement was still expanding rapidly. The capital for the building and other start-up costs were provided by the NSCR and, in line with NSCR policy, the NHS took full responsibility for the hospice's management and running costs. A charitable group called the 'Friends' was established at the same time as the hospice was founded. The Friends committee comprised a number of articulate, middle-class people from the local community, a significant proportion of whom had encountered a personal bereavement at some stage in the past and now wanted to help other people.[23] The role of the committee was envisaged as complementing that of the NHS management: it was the Friends, for example, who were responsible for recruiting, training and supervising all the volunteers who worked in and for the hospice and day care, of whom there were over 200 at the time of my fieldwork. The committee, in addition, organised local fund-raising events such as concerts and fêtes to finance one-off projects such as the building of new staff facilities. The money collected (which included bequests made by some patients in their wills together with donations from families and friends) was also used to provide 'luxuries' for patients such as alcoholic drinks and newspapers. Perhaps most importantly of all, the Friends saw themselves as fulfilling a political function, since they regarded it as their responsibility to promote and safeguard the hospice's long-term aspirations and goals. This situation sometimes brought them into conflict with the NHS management, particularly when the number of beds in the hospice was cut (see below).

The hospice where I carried out my fieldwork was based on the same architectural design as a number of other NHS units established across the country at roughly the same time. It was originally a twenty-five bed unit, divided into four five-bed wards, and five single rooms. The wards were strictly segregated by sex, and were located at the back of the building. The main entrance, located at the front of the building, led directly into a reception area where there was a tea bar staffed by volunteers. At times when the tea bar was closed, family and friends could make themselves drinks and light meals in the visitors' kitchen.[24] The building also contained a small chapel, which doubled up as an overnight room for families of patients who were close to death, and a viewing room where nursing staff took patients after they died and laid their bodies out. Relatives and friends of a deceased patient were given the opportunity to go and view the body in this room; an opportunity which, in practice, only about a half chose to take up. There was a set of double doors at the back of the viewing room, which enabled porters to transfer the corpse straight through the side of the building to the mortuary,[25] rather than having to wheel it through the main entrance.

Some alterations had been made to the hospice building by the time I conducted fieldwork there in 1995. The previous year, the hospice management closed permanently six of the beds after the Health Commission (the 'purchasers') decided to allocate a larger proportion of its palliative care budget to primary care services. The bed cutbacks can be understood within the context of the broader trends highlighted in the previous section, which have led to a shift in hospice provision away from inpatient to home care services and which I discuss in more detail in Chapter 4. One of the five-bed wards had subsequently been converted into a day room, where patients and visitors could congregate and socialise with one another. In addition, one of the single rooms had been converted into a smoking room. Staff decided to use the room for this purpose because they believed that, if patients could smoke in their own homes, they also had a right to do so within the hospice; albeit within a confined space.[26] A diagram of the design and layout of the hospice at the time of my fieldwork is contained in Appendix A.

The building's design, with its emphasis upon open wards and shared spaces, was clearly in line with the hospice ideology of an open confrontation with death. The single rooms were often allocated to middle-class patients (see Chapter 5) and also to patients who had young children (as the nursing staff pointed out, young children were likely to disturb the other patients in the wards because they could be noisy). Hospice staff had, however, also developed an informal practice of moving patients into side rooms if they became paranoid and/or confused, or if there were severe problems with body odours. This practice, as I highlight in later chapters, served as a means by which patients' suffering could be sequestered even within the hospice building.

As in the hospice movement in general, the hospice where I conducted research catered principally for patients with advanced cancer, although a small number of patients with other illnesses such as multiple sclerosis (MS), motor neurone disease (MND) and AIDS were also included in the remit.[27] Patient admissions were divided by staff into four broad and often overlapping categories: those needing 'respite care', a social admission enabling family and other informal carers to have a break from caring for the patient at home; those needing 'pain control'; those needing 'symptom control' (common symptoms included nausea and violent vomiting, chronic incontinence and fungating tumours); and those needing 'terminal care'. Approximately one-third of all patients were admitted to the hospice for terminal care. Other patients returned home, but were often re-admitted at a later stage in their illness and deterioration.

My fieldwork occurred during a particularly notable period of transition and change, since shortly after the study started a further three beds were cut by the NHS managers. The managers' concern to improve the efficiency and cost-effectiveness of the hospice led to increasing pressure being placed upon staff to discharge patients at the earliest possible opportunity and to refill the beds immediately.[28] These changes had a substantial impact upon working practices within the hospice, with staff expected to discharge patients whenever possible after a one or two week period of stay; sometimes, in their opinion, inappropriately.[29] In addition, as I examine further in Chapter 4, the bed cutbacks affected the types of patients who were admitted to the hospice, with bed shortages making it necessary for staff to prioritise what they considered the most pressing and urgent cases. Respite admissions, particularly for non-cancer patients, were substantially curtailed and, for reasons which will also be examined in Chapter 4, the highest priority was generally accorded to patients requiring symptom control.

The day care service

As indicated above, day care services began to be established in various parts of the country after the initial drive to set up hospice inpatient units had lost momentum. Like home care services, the setting up of day care facilities can be understood as resulting from a broader shift towards 'care in the community' occurring in state provision at the time (Holland 1984: 3; Brotchie and Hills 1991; Fisher and McDaid 1996: 4). The first purpose-built day hospice was established at St Lukes Hospice, Sheffield, in 1975, and by the time that I began my fieldwork in 1994, over 200 units had been opened within the UK and Ireland.[30] The day care centre where I conducted fieldwork was opened in January 1993 after several years of discussion and planning between the Friends, the Healthcare Trust (the NHS 'provider') and the local Health Commission (the NHS 'purchaser'). It began as a two-year pilot project, located in makeshift premises near the hospice, and received the bulk of its initial running costs from money raised by the Friends. Whilst the service was founded using charitable sources, it was anticipated that the Health Commission would take responsibility for its long-term running costs once the pilot had come to an end (see also Lunt 1985; Taylor 1983). However, in order to secure permanent funding from the Health Commission, day care had to demonstrate its viability and worth by means of a formal evaluation, designed to monitor the progress of the service and to assess its achievements against its stated aims and objectives. It was at this delicate moment that I came to be involved.

Like other similar services set up across the country, day care aimed to cater for patients with advanced diseases (predominantly cancer) for whom no further active treatment aimed at a cure was being offered, and was principally targeted at those patients who had 'reached that stage in their illness where they are "beginning to lose ground", [but] not such an advanced stage as to make attendance at an in-patient unit more appropriate'.[31] This phase of a patient's illness is often seen as one associated with specific social and emotional difficulties both for them and their family. As the authors of a book written for palliative care professionals suggest:

> For those patients whose disease is life threatening and in-
> curable, many adjustments have to be made to their life-
> styles. They are often too incapacitated to pursue their
> usual routines and hobbies, and quite often they and their
> families are left stunned by the situation. It is for those

patients who are not actually dying, but whose ability to fulfil their usual roles is compromised, that referral to a day care unit is indicated.

(Fisher and McDaid 1996: 4)

The formal aims of day care therefore pay great attention to readjustment and rehabilitation; the goal being to enable patients to return to a normal lifestyle (Fisher and McDaid 1996: 6; Hockley and Mowatt 1996: 13).[32] This objective was clearly evident in the Operational Policy of the service where I conducted fieldwork, from which the following extracts have been drawn. One of day care's stated goals was to help patients adjust to the diagnosis of life-threatening disease by 'providing information to enable the patients and their carers to make informed choices'. In addition, a range of therapeutic activities was planned to assist patients in making adjustments 'to changed circumstances and/or loss of independence' brought about by their illness and deterioration, 'and to cope with the implications of these changes'. The various therapeutic activities on offer included group work, facilitated by the staff, to encourage patients 'to share their feelings with others with a similar diagnosis'; creative activities such as painting, embroidery, woodwork and tapestry to help patients gain a new sense of 'achievement, of pride and self worth'; and complementary therapies such as relaxation and aromatherapy to 'aid sleep, reduce stress and anxiety and relieve pain'. All of the activities provided were intended to 'promote physical and psychological well being', and hence to encourage patients to regain a sense of confidence, independence and autonomy, which in turn would enable them 'to return to their normal way of life as soon as possible'.[33] As I examine in Chapter 2, however, whilst this stage in a patient's illness and deterioration was indeed associated with a significant transition, it was not in the way that was envisaged in the Operational Policy. Consequently, the actual needs experienced by patients were often very different from those which the day care service originally formally set out to address.[34]

The rehabilitative focus of day care was also evident in the length of time patients were entitled to attend the service. Like the majority of other services set up across the country, patients were officially limited to an eight-week 'package' of therapy and psycho-social support (patients normally attended for one day each week), after which their discharge back into 'the community' was anticipated.

The day care service where I conducted fieldwork was open three days each week, and catered for a group of up to eight patients on any one day. Whilst some elderly patients did attend day care, the majority of patients were under sixty and some were in their early thirties; it was believed that younger patients, in particular, would benefit from the service's rehabilitative focus. An occupational therapist was appointed as the day care team leader.[35] Her role was to oversee the day-to-day running of the service; to formulate care plans with patients; and to co-ordinate the various therapeutic and rehabilitative therapies offered within the centre. She was supported by a nurse with special training in massage and relaxation techniques. The nurse was also available to provide patients with advice and information on practical matters such as diet and medication. These two trained members of staff were assisted by a plethora of volunteers (typically two volunteers were on duty at any one time), who had a facilitating and back-up role. They were responsible for setting up and clearing the room at the beginning and end of the day, preparing and serving food and refreshments to patients, assisting those patients with poor mobility, and running errands for the staff. At the time of my fieldwork, all the volunteers working in day care were women although, apparently, one man had worked for the service regularly in the past (the volunteers working in the hospice were also predominantly women). Most volunteers came from middle-class backgrounds, and the majority were in their fifties or early sixties.[36]

My opportunity to conduct fieldwork in day care arose after I was invited to assist with the evaluation, in particular to contribute to its qualitative aspects. As a result, I was asked to observe and participate in the day care Steering Group. This group comprised representatives from the Health Commission, the Healthcare Trust and the Friends, and was set up to oversee the planning and implementation of the evaluation, as well as to make policy decisions and recommendations concerning the future running and financing of the service. My participation in the Steering Group thus created a valuable opportunity to study day care from a different angle from that provided by my participant observation study (i.e. from the top down). This participation, as we shall see further in Chapter 2, drew my attention to a significant discrepancy between the formal goals and objectives of the service – namely the rehabilitative focus discussed above – and an informal model of care which had gradually evolved within the day care setting, through the input and interactions of patients, staff and volunteers.

Whilst my study of day care concentrates principally upon the impact patients' diagnosis and deterioration had upon their sense of self, combined with the various ways in which patients, staff and volunteers sought to negate the debasing effects of illness, the long-term impact of the evaluation will also be considered: significantly, it constituted an arena in which the formal and informal models of care came into direct confrontation with one another for the first time.

Clearly, by conducting fieldwork in both day care and the hospice, I was able to observe patients' experiences of loss of self at two different moments in their illness and deterioration; moments also intersected by the distinctive cultures of the day care and hospice institutions, together with the broader social context within which these institutions were located. Conducting fieldwork in both settings created opportunities for comparison as well as allowing lines of continuity to be traced. It often proved to be the case, for instance, that patients I originally met in day care were later encountered during my fieldwork in the hospice. Such patients, though much weaker and more lethargic, often had a story to tell about what had happened during the period between being discharged from the first setting and admitted into the second.

Entering 'the field': methods of access and data collection

Setting up a viable fieldwork project is a challenge with which all anthropologists have to contend. In my case, however, the very nature of the research I chose to conduct – a study of patients who were dying – created what initially seemed to be a whole series of potentially impenetrable barriers. Such barriers stemmed in part from the supposedly taboo nature of death and dying in the UK, but were reinforced by my status as a non-medical professional who wished to conduct research within a medical setting. Indeed, medical professionals are notoriously very protective of their patients; dying patients, however, are thought to be at a particularly vulnerable and fragile stage in their lives: a phenomenon which has led some professionals to question whether such patients should be included in research at all (see Kritjanson *et al.* 1994). It is perhaps not too surprising, therefore, that many of my early attempts to set up a research project were unsuccessful: most of the hospital and hospice professionals I contacted did not respond to the letters I wrote outlining my research interests and requesting a meeting. Whilst I am certain that their hectic work schedules were major contributory factors in this regard, it is also very likely that the difficulties I encountered were at least partly attributable to the nature of the research I had chosen to conduct.[37]

The opportunity to conduct fieldwork in the day care service thus came about as much by luck as any other factor. I originally wrote to the day care team leader expressing an interest in learning more about the goals and objectives of the service, together with the views and experiences of patients who used it. My letter, as it turned out, arrived at a perfect time. As I have already described above, the NHS Trust (the 'providers') were in the process of implementing an evaluation to monitor the service's progress and benefits, and the NHS Trust's Head of Research and Development (R&D) was looking for someone with a research interest in palliative care to help out with this project.[38] In a meeting involving myself, the Head of R&D and day care's NHS Trust manager, it was agreed that I could conduct a participant observation study within day care and use any insights and material I gained both for the evaluation and for my own research purposes. I was also given permission to conduct unstructured and semi-structured interviews with patients and their family and friends (provided patients had given their prior consent), as well as with day care's staff and volunteers.

The bulk of time in this meeting was actually spent deliberating over how I should label and present myself to patients within day care. It was clear from the outset that patients should be fully informed about my research, but we also agreed that my presence within day care had the potential to be too cumbersome and distracting to patients and staff alike if I went in solely in a research capacity. As we all agreed, I needed to be in a role that would give me a legitimate reason to spend large amounts of time within day care, without my presence necessarily having to affect the internal dynamics taking place there. A decision was thus reached that I should work in a volunteer capacity as this would allow me considerable contact with patients (for example, serving them food and refreshments), as well as enabling me to work directly alongside paid staff and other volunteers. Although this seemed to be the most viable option at the time, we were, nevertheless, somewhat concerned that patients might find it too confusing if I wore two hats simultaneously: they might, for instance, be uncertain whether I was interacting with them in a 'volunteer' or 'research' capacity on any particular occasion. It is interesting, therefore, that I did not encounter any obvious problems with how I should present myself once I actually began my fieldwork. The reason is quite simple: as I discuss further in Chapter 2, in their day-to-day interactions with one another, day care participants avoided using any labels or other criteria which would differentiate 'carers' (staff and volunteers) from the 'cared for' (patients). Whilst staff always explained my research interests and involvement with the evaluation to patients, and I performed volunteer duties alongside other volunteers, patients chose not to label or perceive me either as a 'researcher' or as a 'volunteer'. Rather, I became 'Julia', a member of the 'day care family', who was placed on an equal footing with all the other participants.

All of day care's patients consented to participate in the research both for the evaluation and also for this book. Their response to the research was, overall, extremely positive. Part of the reason for their enthusiasm stemmed from the fact that they valued coming to day care, and hence they hoped that I would be able to use my observations to help to secure long-term funding for the service. (In this regard, I felt I carried a heavy responsibility on my shoulders throughout the time I was conducting the study.) Yet patients' willingness to help with the research was also, I suggest, sympto-matic of the sense of isolation that many of them experienced. Several patients commented that they found it helpful to share their experiences of their illness with me, because I was one of the few people who seemed comfortable and willing to listen to them, pitting me in contrast to their own family and friends. One woman added that it was 'very comforting' that I cared about them all sufficiently to want to do research in day care in the first place. I received a very similar response from members of patients' families who participated in unstructured interviews.[39] My interviews with patients' main carers drew my attention to the fact that these people often felt equally, if not more, isolated than the patients themselves: clearly a patient's illness and deterioration could have a marked impact upon a whole network of people.

My fieldwork in day care began at the end of April 1994 and I visited the centre regularly until the end of September 1994, by which time the evaluation had been written up and presented to the Health Commission. During these five months, I was able to observe and interview roughly forty patients in total, together with twelve family members. I also returned to the centre for a brief period of follow-up research approximately ten months later to explore the long-term impact of the evaluation.

Because I had developed a good rapport with day care's staff and patients, it actually proved to be comparatively easy to set up a second project within the hospice. The hospice staff had heard positive reports about my fieldwork in day care and, consequently, were willing to allow me to conduct an ethnographic study within their own institution. The general consensus of opinion was that, since I had already shown that I was capable of interacting with patients in a careful and sensitive manner, I would be extremely unlikely to upset their own patients. Yet, at a meeting set up to discuss my fieldwork arrangements, it also became evident that staff's willingness to allow me to conduct research in the hospice stemmed partly from the fact that, at the time, they were preoccupied with several practical and ethical issues relating to their own working practices. It was proposed, therefore, that I might be able to help them to address these matters through my own research.

One of the concerns presented to me centred upon the very limited use made by patients of the hospice's new day room. As I described earlier, six beds in the hospice had been permanently cut some months previously, and one of the five-bed wards had subsequently been converted into a day room. Although staff had objected to the bed cutbacks, they had hoped patients would use this new room to socialise with one another, to watch television and to participate in relaxation sessions and other craft and therapeutic activities supervised by the hospice's occupational therapist. In spite of considerable encouragement from staff and volunteers, however, the majority of patients preferred to remain in the wards or in their side rooms. Staff suggested, therefore, that I might be able identify the reasons why patients were so reluctant to use the day room and recommend ways in which their participation could be increased.

Hospice staff had also begun to question their practice of keeping dying patients in communal wards after two patients in quick succession had requested a discharge as a result of witnessing the death of another patient in the same room as them. They had also received a letter of complaint from a widower who felt strongly that his wife should have been placed in a side room when she was dying. He suggested that he had felt unable to express his grief at the time of his wife's death because he did not want to upset the other patients and visitors present in the ward. Staff thus hoped that I would be able to befriend patients and obtain their views on whether they found it helpful or unhelpful to see other patients die beside them. The general consensus of opinion was that patients would be more comfortable confiding in me because I was not a member of staff.

Whilst, in practice, the staff's interest in my research began to fade fairly rapidly once the novelty of my being in the hospice had started to wear off, I continued to pay attention to these particular issues during my fieldwork. As I examine in later chapters, both issues constituted a dilemma for hospice staff because each, in similar ways, encapsulated the difficulties of aligning the 'rhetorics of individuality' embedded within the hospice philosophy of care with the realities of how personhood is lived and lost in everyday life.

Kritjanson *et al.* (1994), de Raeve (1994) and Randall and Downie (1996) have all written specifically about the practical, moral and ethical problems involved in conducting research amongst palliative care populations. As Kritjanson *et al.* suggest, dying patients become easily fatigued, are likely to experience some degree of physical discomfort, and also suffer in response to their knowledge of impending death, the stress of settling their affairs, and the emotional strains of dealing with family members (1994: 11). It was largely for reasons such as these that direct observation and informal conversation techniques were used very extensively as methods of data collection in the hospice, whereas formal interviews were only employed extremely rarely. Formal interviews not only seemed to be too obtrusive to many patients and their families; in a substantial number of instances they simply were not viable. Some patients, for example, were heavily sedated during their stay in the hospice, whilst others experienced changes in their mental state, such as becoming very paranoid or confused. It was, of course, impossible to interview a patient in a coma.

I worked as an 'in-house' volunteer within the hospice because this particular role enabled me to have substantial and regular contact with patients and their visitors in the wards, side rooms and other communal areas within the building. The role of in-house volunteer encompassed a wide range of patient related and practical tasks. The former included duties such as befriending and talking to patients, relatives and visitors; serving pre-lunch drinks to patients; and escorting patients to hospital appointments. The latter involved such things as stripping and making beds, arranging flowers and washing patients' personal laundry (for a comprehensive list of the in-house volunteer duties see Appendix B). I often found that performing a practical task, such as making a bed, gave me an ideal excuse to enter a ward and make observations in situations when it might otherwise have been too awkward and obtrusive to have a researcher present: for instance, when one of the patients in the ward had just died.

In addition to being allowed to move freely within the wards, side rooms and other communal parts of the building, hospice staff also gave me permission to sit in on their hand-overs, multi-disciplinary team meetings, and case conferences. The hand-overs took place in the nurses' office and occurred each time a new group of nurses came on duty. Their purpose was to update nurses on new admissions and any changes that had occurred in patients' conditions since they were last on duty. The multi-disciplinary meetings were held once a week (on a Monday morning) and included the hospice doctors; the senior nursing sister; representatives from the nursing teams; the chaplain; the social worker; the counsellor; the occupational therapist; the physiotherapist; and (occasionally) the volunteer co-ordinator. Each patient was discussed in detail during the meeting and the team made joint decisions about the types of medical and psycho-social care that should be offered to him or her (on some occasions, the multi-disciplinary team also decided to extend emotional and social care to a member of a patient's family, by offering them, for example, a counselling session). The multi-disciplinary meetings were also the forum in which staff decided if, and when, it would be possible for patients to be discharged. Case conferences were held approximately once a month and were set up to enable staff to discuss a patient they had found particularly difficult and distressing to care for in the hospice. The staff hoped that they would be able to improve the care they offered to other patients if they reflected upon and learnt from cases where they felt they had 'failed'.

Whenever possible, patients were informed by staff about my research and given the option of 'opting out' of any observations I made. In cases where a patient was admitted in a coma, or was suffering from confusion, the consent of his or her relatives was obtained instead. Whilst some patients were genuinely very supportive of, and interested in, my study, many maintained a polite, but detached, disinterest; a situation which pitted them in contrast to day care patients. Such a phenomenon, as I explore further in later chapters, stemmed largely from the fact that, by the time patients had been admitted to the hospice, many had become very disengaged from all events taking place around them. Only one hospice patient, however, actually asked to be excluded from any observations I made. Consequently, with the exception of this one patient, the observations developed in this book include the entire hospice population during the fieldwork period. In the ten months I worked in the hospice, I came into contact with roughly 280 different patients, together with a similar number of family members, friends and other visitors. Approximately 200 deaths occurred within the hospice during the period that I was there.

The practical and ethical difficulties I experienced whilst conducting fieldwork in the hospice were, in many respects, considerably more complex than those encountered within day care.[40] One of my major and repeated concerns centred upon the issue of informed consent: I became acutely aware that, just because patients had given their consent to be included in my research on their admission to the hospice, such consent could not necessarily be taken for granted in my later encounters with them. It is precisely because patients experienced a loss of self as their diseases progressed that I could not necessarily assume that a patient I observed in the final stages approaching death was necessarily the *same person* who had originally given their consent. Yet to have attempted to continuously re-solicit consent from patients would also have raised a number of practical and moral difficulties: patients could, and did, become very anxious and afraid as they became more unwell. A further dilemma stemmed from the fact that, in order to make observations for my research in an unobtrusive fashion I had, in a sense, to become a part of the institution I was studying: hence my working in the hospice in a volunteer capacity. The one obvious worry I had about conducting fieldwork in this way is that it is extremely likely that, on some occasions at least, patients shared personal information with me because they perceived me first and foremost as a volunteer, quite possibly forgetting that I was also collecting observations for my own research. I have tried to keep concerns such as these in mind in the pages that follow and have quoted patients selectively. All patients, however, have been included in the general themes and trends highlighted and analysed in this study.

Whilst staff were also aware of the complexities just outlined, the feedback they gave me at the end of my fieldwork was, overall, very positive. Their positive attitude stemmed in large part from the fact that my research had not caused any obvious upset to patients or disruption to their own routines. Staff in fact pointed to a number of benefits that had been gained by having me present in the hospice in a participant observer capacity: they all, for example, could think of instances when patients and their families had found it helpful and comforting to have me around on a regular basis to talk to and spend time with. Nursing staff and other volunteers had also found it very useful to have an extra person to help out in the wards at times when they were busy. Some members of staff, however, were more ambivalent about my being allowed to attend their own meetings. A few suggested that there had been occasions when the presence of a researcher had inhibited them from talking openly of feelings of impotence and anguish they experienced as a result of caring for some patients.

The research conducted for this book was approved by the Local Research Ethics Committee of the Health Authority to which day care and the hospice belonged. The identities of all persons mentioned in this book have been protected through the use of pseudonyms. For obvious reasons, I have also chosen not to disclose the exact location of the hospice and day care service where I conducted fieldwork. Staff in both settings were given, and have taken up, the opportunity to read earlier versions of this work, and I am extremely grateful for their help in clarifying some of the factual details outlined in the pages that follow.

The 'typicality' of the research sample

One further thing to comment and reflect upon in this chapter is the 'typicality' of the patients I had access to during fieldwork. Not only did the vast majority of patients I encountered have cancer, there are some grounds for arguing that these particular patients were in certain senses atypical of cancer patients as a whole. As I have already indicated above, the hospice received considerably more referrals than staff were able to accommodate.[41] Consequently, staff had no choice but to give priority to what they regarded as being the most pressing and urgent cases which, in practice, were often patients who experienced particularly distressing *bodily* symptoms such as chronic diarrhoea or violent and repeated vomiting. It is extremely unlikely, therefore, that I observed a random selection of patients in this setting. On the contrary, it appears that the hospice had become an enclave for some of the most distressing cancer deaths.

A particularly distinctive feature of the hospice, and to a lesser extent of day care, furthermore, is their stereotype of being places where one goes to die, a stereotype which many patients were aware of. It was fairly common for patients to describe the hospice using phrases such as 'the point of no return' or 'the death house'. Because patients normally had to give their consent before they were admitted to the hospice (and day care), it is very likely that they constituted a self-selecting sample to some extent. As staff pointed out, patients who were in denial about their illness, and those who were particularly afraid of death, often refused to be admitted, preferring to receive treatment and care in a hospital setting instead. It is not surprising, therefore, that most of the patients I encountered during fieldwork appeared to have an open awareness of their illness; in fact, many hospice patients were surprisingly forthright in talking about death.

Regrettably, I am not in a position to comment upon ethnic differences in this book because the hospice and day care service where I conducted research were located in a part of England with very small ethnic minority populations. In fact, I only encountered one patient who was obviously from an ethnic minority group during my fieldwork (a man, originally from Singapore, who was a devout Buddhist). The two services described in this book were not actually that atypical in this regard. The small amount of research conducted to date suggests that there is a very low uptake of hospice and other specialist services by black and ethnic minority populations in the UK, even in areas where such groups comprise a significant proportion of the population (see Eve *et al.* 1997). The one report specifically addressing the social reasons behind this phenomenon makes the point that people from ethnic minority groups often emigrate back to their country of origin in later life and, consequently, die there. It also highlights the need for more information to be made available to ethnic minority patients and their carers, because they are not currently being advised about palliative care services. The report, in addition, makes the more general observation that ethnic groups feel alienated from mainstream systems of health care delivery because of the failure of these agencies to accommodate and understand their cultural and religious requirements (Hill and Penso 1995; see also Smaje and Field 1997; Gunaratnam 1997). Since ethnic minority patients were largely absent in the hospice and day care, it is not that surprising that the vast majority of patients who described themselves as 'religious' were from Judeo-Christian backgrounds.[42]

It should also be noted that the vast majority of patients admitted to, and attending, day care on a long-term basis were from working-class backgrounds. As I indicated earlier, day care was marketed to patients as being a service which catered for groups. It is fairly likely, therefore, that middle-class patients felt alienated from this sort of environment because of the value they placed on their own privacy (see Chapter 5). Indeed, one of the middle-class patients I spoke to in the hospice suggested that she had been put off going to day care because she imagined it as being somewhat akin to a 'working-class cancer club'. There was, however, a much more balanced mix of patients from middle-class and working-class backgrounds in the hospice,[43] although, as we shall see, class segregations were also very evident *within* this setting: middle-class patients, as a general rule, opted for, and were allocated, single rooms within the hospice building, whereas working-class patients preferred to stay in wards. As I examine further at the end of Chapter 5, one of the most surprising observations made during my research was that, even after patients had lost many attributes of self due to their illness and deterioration, class appeared to be the one aspect of *themselves* which many retained more or less right up until the point of death.

It is also helpful to flag up at this stage that gender will not feature prominently as a theme of observation in the main sections of this book, because gendered differences did not appear to be particularly noticeable amongst the patients with whom I worked. The possible reasons for this phenomenon will be also explored at the end of Chapter 5.

The organisation of the book

This book is organised into different topics and themes divided roughly by chapter. In Chapter 2, the research conducted in day care is described. The first part of the chapter explores patients' anecdotal accounts of their lives outside the day care setting with attention paid to the factors that precipitated their admission. Patients generally entered this arena at a time when their public and private worlds had been shattered by the social perceptions of their illness, and by a sea of *irreversible* changes that had occurred in their interactions with the people around them. Many had become estranged from their networks of interpersonal relationships, partly because of the stigmatising effects of their illness and the physical deterioration that had ensued, but also, as this chapter uncovers, because their temporal perceptions had moved out of synchrony with those of family and friends.

The second part of the chapter explores the various informal strategies employed by patients, staff and volunteers within day care to appropriate the setting and to convert it, as the chapter's title suggests, into a 'safe retreat'. Within this 'safe retreat', patients claimed that they both felt, and were treated like 'normal people', a situation which stood in stark contrast to their experiences outside the day care setting. The day care 'safe retreat' is thus interpreted as being a space within which a patient's self could be successfully sustained.

Chapters 3 and 4 move away from the day care setting to focus upon the experiences of patients admitted to the hospice. Hospice patients were generally significantly more unwell than their day care counterparts: indeed, a significant proportion of patients were actually admitted to the hospice to die. It was during the final stages of their deterioration, as both chapters highlight in different ways, that a patient's body enters 'centre stage'; a patient's bodily deterioration often had an absolutely fundamental, non-negotiable impact upon his or her self.

Chapter 3 examines the transition from 'subject' to 'object' that occurred as patients lost the bodily ability to act as the agents of their actions and intentions. It begins by outlining the recent sociological and anthropological literature on the lived body and embodiment: the chapter aims to show that these approaches have not in fact succeeded in bringing the body as a material, physically experienced phenomenon fully into social analysis. The chapter focuses specifically upon the experiences of 'high-dependency' patients who received care within the hospice and analyses the observation that, as their bodily strength and mobility deteriorated significantly, many appeared to experience a tangential dislocation and loss of self. A phenomenological approach is developed to explore the interdependency of body, self, space and time experienced by these patients: as patients' bodies became reduced to an inert state, their conceptions of space and time also appeared to become progressively bounded and static.

This chapter also highlights and examines the intersubjective impact a patient's loss of mobility had upon family and friends involved with his or her immediate bodily care. Observations of patient–carer interactions are used to indicate that, in the process of providing a dependent patient with 'total body care', the patient's body may become, to some extent, assimilated into, and merged with, a carer's own sense of self. This material not only provides comprehensive ethnographic support for the argument that illnesses affect social networks rather than individuals, it is also fed into a more general critique of anthropological (and other) models of the 'Western' person/self.

The final part of Chapter 3 develops and analyses the observation that, by the time a patient had reached a point close to death, the hospice often seemed to be left caring not for a person, but a mere body. Such material is used to provide a critique of the hospice movement's ideological goal of enabling patients to 'live until they die', due to its failure to take account of the 'bodily realities of dying'. This critique is extended through an exploration of the hospice's practice of keeping dying patients in communal wards and of sedating those who became paranoid or confused.

Chapter 4 develops lines of enquiry opened up in the previous chapter by focusing upon a special case of loss of bodily autonomy: the loss of control of the body's physical boundaries. The physically bounded body, as this chapter indicates, is another aspect of embodiment which is central to personhood in modern 'Western' contexts; a feature of person and self, furthermore, which only fully becomes evident as such after it has been lost.

The chapter begins by examining why, within a prevailing cultural and historical climate of economic cutbacks, and the associated shift towards the care of dying patients at home, the hospice gave priority to patients requiring 'symptom control'. By showing that it was not dying as such, but rather certain specific types of demise that were to be found within the hospice, this chapter highlights the difficulties of continuing to use homogeneous categories such as 'the dying patient' and 'the dying process' to discuss the marginalisation of patients within the physical spaces of hospices and other similar institutions. Such categories are challenged by pointing to the importance of focusing upon the body of the patient, and the disease processes taking place within it and upon its surfaces, in order to understand why some patients were sequestered within the hospice whereas others were not. Through the exploration of a number of case studies, it is suggested that patients were admitted to the hospice not because they were dying *per se*, but rather because of the ways in which their disease spread was destroying, not only their ability to act, but also the *physical* boundaries of their bodies. The chapter also employs both historical and cross-cultural material to explain why the sequestration of the unbounded body is deemed both appropriate, and necessary, within contexts such as contemporary England.

In Chapter 5, the body is allowed to recede temporarily into the background to enable a second, related way in which patients experienced a loss of self to be explored: a loss of self that stemmed from a loss of interpersonal relationships. The experiences of both day care and hospice patients are drawn upon to highlight the various ways in which patients had become progressively dislodged and disconnected from their networks of interpersonal relationships as their illnesses progressed. Such patients are shown to have experienced a form of 'social death' that occurred prior to their physical deaths; a situation which, in its most extreme form, prompted requests for euthanasia and/or the refusal of all food and medication. Whilst a number of hospice patients 'lived after their time', this chapter also examines the experiences of a small group of patients who encountered the opposite problem: that their deaths were going to dislodge them from their relational networks too prematurely. The chapter explores a number of strategies requested by these particular patients, and employed by hospice staff, to sustain their selfhood to a point as close as possible to that of their physical demise.

Whilst relationships are thus shown to be absolutely central to conceptions and experiences of selfhood in 'Western' contexts, the chapter goes on to implicate patients' bodily deterioration directly and indirectly in processes which led to their social deaths. Observations of this type are used to critique the literature on 'the body' for its general failure to examine and locate bodies fully within the context of relationships: Goffman's work (1959, 1963) is shown to be only a partial corrective in this regard. Giddens' (1991, 1993) work on the role of intimacy and emotions in the making of the modern 'Western' self through social connections is similarly critiqued for its essentially 'disembodied' perspective.

The final chapter begins by drawing together the themes and issues discussed in previous chapters through an examination of why many patients seemed more distressed by the ways in which they were actually dying than they were by the prospect of death as such. Cross-cultural and historical data are employed to suggest that the disinvestment of person/self that, in the 'West', occurs prior to physical death, may be reversed in cultures where death is conceived as a liminal phase leading into another form of existence. The chapter also explores some of the implications of the book's findings for the future of palliative care, and examines the somewhat contentious role that the modern hospice movement plays in contemporary debates on euthanasia and physician-assisted suicide. It closes with some brief reflections upon the theoretical contributions of the study.

2

DAY CARE

A safe retreat

Day care: a safe retreat

This is our place, our safe retreat,
Where each week we come to meet.
We meet to share with each our care,
It's good for us to be just here.

We know that sickness is no easy thing,
Whatever the sickness, or if we can't win.
We think that cancer socks the lot,
Because that's what we suffer, – so what–

–For too–
There are many people who suffer pain,
Many who will never walk again,
Many who will never see the light of day,
Many too, who will have no word to say.

Many who will not see the chorus of dawn,
Others wonder, why am I forlorn.
Others who will not give way to their plight,
Others show courage and keep up their fight.

We know we have to fight to win,
To triumph over this cancer thing.
Some may know there is no cure,
But of one thing we are very sure.

Our healing will come from within,
Peace of heart and mind will win.
And when we meet here in this place,
We thank God for another day of grace.
(Poem written by a former day care patient and
used here with her kind permission)

The objectives of day care are to rehabilitate where possible, improve the quality of life of patients and to provide a 'stepping-stone' to more appropriate local agencies where these exist.

The aim of day care is to reach people early in the palliative phase of their disease and enable them to return to their normal way of life as soon as possible. Some adjustments may be necessary; day care provides the information and assistance required to make choices and reach decisions and allows patients to exercise control over their lives.
(Formal aims and objectives of day care – extracts from the Operational Policy)

Introduction

In Chapter 1 I outlined the formal aims and objectives of the day care pilot, highlighting in particular the strong emphasis given to rehabilitation, premised upon the idea of relatively short 'packages' of care offered to each individual patient. Yet if the formal goals of day care are juxtaposed with the poem above, it becomes evident that the service was perceived and valued by its participants in a very different way. Far from being seen as a rehabilitative stepping-stone, day care, as the poem's title aptly suggests, was valued as a 'safe retreat' or, as another patient described it, as 'a safe haven'. Patients frequently suggested that day care constituted the one space available to them in which they felt that they could 'be themselves', 'live with their cancer', or, as one woman put it, 'return to a normal life'.

Furthermore, when patients reflected upon their experiences outside the day care setting, it became apparent that the self-identities they enacted in day care differed substantially from those in their own homes. In day care, patients were often active and engaged; outside day care their lives tended to be characterised by increasing isolation, dependency and disengagement.

In this chapter I suggest that, in response to patients' actual, experienced needs, an informal model of care had evolved within day care which differed noticeably from the service's formal goals and objectives. The formal rehabilitative ethos of day care could not have worked in practice, because of the impossibility of 'rehabilitating' or altering the context into which the patients had to return: the cultural setting outside of day care. Consequently, day care's patients could only be 'rehabilitated' within its immediate confines.

In the ethnographic discussion and analysis below, a number of complex interactional processes emerge through which the day care setting was appropriated by patients, staff and volunteers in their day-to-day interactions, and thereby converted into an 'alternative reality';[1] a 'new social world'. This 'alternative reality' provided an arena, in contrast to the world outside, in which the patients were able to realise and sustain a comparatively stable sense of self; it permitted a preservation of their personhood, in spite of the experiences of loss and of bodily deterioration which occurred in their lives outside the day care setting. The construction of day care as a 'safe haven', as we shall see, was dependent not only upon the day care participants managing the space and events taking place within the immediate setting, but also on them regulating and mediating various activities occurring at its boundaries.

Characteristics of patients admitted to day care: disintegration and loss of self

> The needs of patients with life-threatening conditions are *quite unique*. They have a future that cannot be mapped out plus a disease which is likely to cause rapid deterioration in their physical and mental capacities. Consequently, many patients feel *extremely isolated*.
>
> (Jackie, Macmillan nurse; emphasis added)

This section explores patients' anecdotal accounts of the ways in which a diagnosis of incurable illness, coupled with the impact of their encroaching disease, affected their lives outside the day care setting. These accounts provide a necessary context for understanding why the 'alternative reality' generated within day care developed in the ways it did and, furthermore, why the informal model of care came to diverge so radically from the formal goals and objectives of the service.

Jackie, whose words are quoted above, was one of the three Macmillan nurses responsible for the majority of referrals to day care.[2] Her comments touch on a theme which will form the focal point of observation and analysis in this section: how patients' experiences of their illness and deterioration led to a debasement of self and to a disengagement from the 'matrix of social relations' (Moore 1994: 31) within which they were previously located. As we shall see, patients were often subjected to social isolation – imposed and/or self-imposed – not only because of the loss of mobility stemming from their physical deterioration, but also as a result of the stigmatising effects of their illness. In addition, a number of patients suffered from what Jackie, on another occasion, intuitively termed 'a sense of isolation with their disease'. Patients became increasingly estranged from their networks of interpersonal ties because their temporal frameworks, their 'future that cannot be mapped out', ceased to synchronise with those of family and friends. Consequently, many patients found themselves in a state of being with which other people were unable to identify. The isolation, disengagement and physical dependency that patients experienced led to a debasement and erosion of their personhood; to a loss of self, which the 'alternative reality' enacted within day care served to reinstate.

House-bound patients

Many patients at this stage in their illness suffered from both physical and social isolation as a result of the debilitative effects of their cancer, and the consequent impact this had upon their mobility and autonomy. The spread of cancer to the bones and lungs, in particular, resulted in physical weakness and lethargy, causing some patients to become wheelchair bound, while others had to use a walking frame to cover any significant distance. As a consequence, most patients had to give up an independent lifestyle and some had become house-bound. House-bound patients, in particular, confronted substantial difficulties in generating and maintaining social contacts and, in cases where the patient lived alone, the social isolation that ensued could be very severe.

Fred, a man in his eighties, was a good case in point. He originally developed cancer of the prostate, but by the time he was admitted to day care the cancer had spread to his lungs. He also had a heart condition. Fred could thus only manage minimal physical exertion before he became extremely out of breath. His deterioration had been comparatively recent; until about six weeks prior to his admission he had been able to walk without assistance. Now he required a wheelchair to travel any distance. As he lived alone and had no family or friends living locally to take him out, he had become house-bound.

Fred frequently complained that he felt like 'an animal trapped in a cage' when he was at home. However, the full extent of his isolation, and the impact this had upon him, only became fully apparent when I was asked to collect him from his house and escort him to day care in a taxi. I had to enter his house through an unlocked back door because Fred was too weak to walk over and open his front door. I arrived to find him in a flood of tears sitting on a commode in the middle of his living room. Fred had had an attack of breathlessness shortly before I arrived, and this had temporarily left him too weak to lift himself off the commode. Once he regained his composure, we started to chat. Fred drew my attention to the severely limited amount of space he was able to negotiate and move around within his own home. Now that he could only manage to walk a few paces without assistance, his district nurse had moved his bed downstairs into the living room. A chair had been placed next to the bed, and the commode next to the chair. With effort, Fred could move himself from one piece of furniture to another. As he pointed out, he was confined to about nine square metres of space within his living room.

Fred also complained about his social isolation, which had become especially marked since his physical deterioration.[3] He was no longer able to walk to the pub or to his local pensioners' club, and no-one visited him apart from a neighbour who did his shopping, and a care assistant who came briefly in the mornings and evenings to help him get up and go to bed.

Similarly, Iris, a woman in her seventies, had breast cancer and bone secondaries and could only manage to walk short distances with the aid of a stick. Iris was one of the favourites in day care because she was constantly cheerful and fond of teasing the staff and other patients. However, Iris painted a very different picture of her life at home. There she spent 'endless empty hours vegetating in front of the television'. The monotony of her routine was only broken by visits from her daughter (living locally) who brought her meals. Because she was house-bound, she had lost contact with the small number of her friends who were still alive. The effect on her life was devastating. According to her granddaughter, Iris had 'more or less given up' the last time she was discharged from hospital. In the granddaughter's opinion, Iris' once weekly visits to day care were, 'the only thing that's keeping my gran going. If it wasn't for day care I don't think she'd have a reason for getting out of bed in the mornings.'

Stigmatisation

Social isolation also resulted from the stigmatisation of the patient by others, and the growing sense of alienation that ensued. Patients repeatedly complained that other people had ceased both to see them and to treat them as 'normal', particularly when the progression of their disease (or its treatment) affected their physical appearance. Such a phenomenon is highlighted particularly graphically in anecdotes provided by Anne. Anne's bodily appearance had deteriorated significantly after she became unwell. She originally developed a malignant melanoma, and had brain surgery to remove the tumour, followed by chemotherapy. As a consequence, her hair had become very thin and had not grown back fully where the surgery had been performed. The cancer had also spread to her liver, causing mild jaundice. Due to increasing weakness and lethargy, she had to walk with a stick.

Anne described a number of incidents where friends and other people in her village had started ignoring her, sometimes even avoiding her altogether, after she became 'visibly unwell'. On several occasions, she had been sitting in the front garden at home and neighbours had, 'crossed the street and ignored me completely. … I'm now treated as if my cancer is contagious in some sort of way.' In addition, her best friend had stopped coming round to visit her. When Anne's daughter confronted her about this matter, the friend apparently offered the following explanation:

> I feel she can't do the things she used to do. She doesn't look normal; she doesn't act normal, so I can't talk to her in a normal way. I suppose I've started avoiding her because I don't want to hurt her feelings.

Anne's husband had also made it clear that he was uncomfortable being seen with her in public. He refused to take her into town in her wheelchair because he was worried that he might be spotted by his 'mates'.[4]

It was, indeed, a common complaint amongst day care patients that family and friends were only supportive and attentive on occasions when they 'looked and acted normal'. As one woman, Wendy, dryly remarked: 'On those bad days when I wake up and feel terrible, *and look terrible*, no-one wants to know me' (emphasis added).

It sometimes proved to be the case, however, that a patient's alienation and disengagement from their social networks was also, to some extent, internalised and self-imposed. Jan, for example, had to have a mastectomy after receiving a diagnosis of breast cancer. When the doctors came to operate they discovered that her cancer was so advanced that they had to remove a substantial amount of the muscle from her rib-cage. Jan woke up from her operation to discover that there was only a very thin dressing covering her extensive wound. She lifted up the dressing and found her rib cage totally exposed; she could even see her heart beating underneath it. At the time, Jan claimed that she 'nearly died of fright'. Whilst a skin graft was performed at a later date, the long-term scarification and bodily disfigurement was very severe. The day care nurse, Lucy, confessed that she had difficulty keeping her composure the first time Jan took off her clothes to receive a massage. The impact upon Jan's sense of self was very marked. She told me that she still could not bring herself to look at her 'mutilated body', even though it had been several years now since the operation had been performed. At night she would lie in bed with her night-gown fully buttoned to the top, covered with her bed clothes, no matter how hot it was. As Jan went on to claim, 'I'll never see myself as a woman again'. She did not have a partner at the time, and suggested that she would never allow herself to have a relationship in the future because, 'I don't think I could cope with his rejection on top of my own'.

The experiences of patients such as Anne and Jan can, I suggest, be understood by looking at Goffman's pioneering work on stigma in which he argues that if a person, 'possesses an attribute that makes him [sic] different from others in the category of persons available for him to be. ... He is reduced in our minds from a whole and usual person to a tainted and discounted one' (1963: 12). Amongst the various factors which can lead to stigmatisation, Goffman points to 'abominations of the body – the various physical deformities' (1963: 14). Such an observation also finds support in Davis' recent research on cosmetic surgery. As her study suggests, most people do not have cosmetic surgery out of a desire to be more beautiful (1995: 88). On the contrary, their hope is 'to become unnoticeable', 'to be one of the crowd' (1995: 82), by having a physical characteristic altered which they believe makes them look abnormal (1995: 89).[5]

Temporal isolation

Patients' experience of 'isolation with their disease' is a complex phenomenon to examine and dissect. I often gained the impression, for example, that patients' 'lived experience' of their illness, and the bodily deterioration accompanying it, had eroded and undermined their previously taken-for-granted world-views, thus causing their subjective conceptions of reality to come out of line with those of family and friends. Patients were, it seemed, often drawn into what Charmaz has termed an 'odyssey of self' (1995a: 675), in which their changing and deteriorating bodies had become 'alien terrain', and their 'altered lives' had transported them into 'unfamiliar worlds' where they felt 'estranged' (ibid.; see also Charmaz 1991). It is certainly significant that patients often spoke of receiving more empathy and understanding from one another than from their own (healthy and able-bodied) family and friends. This phenomenon, which I examine in more detail in Chapter 3, was made especially apparent when patients reflected on the ways in which their weakness, lethargy and loss of mobility had affected their lives. As Paul suggested,

> I can't do the things I used to do; I can't do the things I want to do. My family don't understand why I get so angry and upset. ... I suppose taking the dog for a walk, or making a cup of tea isn't that big a deal until you can't do it anymore. ... At least here [referring to the other patients in day care] we all understand each other. After all, we're all in the same boat.

Day care patients frequently used phrases such as 'in the same boat' and 'kindred spirits' to express the subjective world-view they shared with one another, but not with other persons. In this respect, their experiences closely paralleled those of the patients studied by Jackson who attended a chronic pain clinic in the United States. Jackson's patients felt that they belonged to a 'pain-full world' (1994: 218) which others 'could not possibly understand' (ibid.), and, consequently, that they were members of 'a very exclusive club' (1994: 216).

Patients' experience of 'isolation with their disease' became evident, not only in their changing experiences of embodiment, but also in their different sense and perception of time. The diagnosis of incurable cancer often built up walls between patients, their families, and others, leading to a breakdown and conflict in understanding and communication and, in some cases, to what has been termed a 'conspiracy of silence' (Kübler-Ross 1969; Boston and Trezise 1987: 52). This conflict in understanding, as I now go on to illustrate, often stemmed from the fact that patients' conceptions of time (and therefore of themselves in time) had become radically different from that of their family and friends.

My attention was first drawn to the disparate nature of patients' temporal experiences when I conducted an unstructured interview with Karen, a 52-year-old woman with breast cancer, at an early stage in my fieldwork. After we had completed the interview, Karen asked me what had particularly drawn me into wanting to do research in day care. I replied that I had wanted to work in a setting which would put me in close contact with patients who had terminal illnesses. I did not, however, get any further with my explanation because Karen launched into a very fierce attack upon my use of the word 'terminal': 'How dare you use a word like that here! There's something about it that I find quite distasteful.'

Karen went on to explain why I had triggered such an angry response. The previous week she had had to fill out a Department of Social Security form for sickness benefit.[6] One of the questions on this form asked if she had a terminal illness. The form went on to define a terminal illness as meaning the person had a life expectancy of six months or less. Karen's sense of anger then became more understandable: 'How dare they write me off like that! Why use words like "advanced" or "terminal" at all? They take away your right to hope.'

What this encounter between Karen and me served to highlight is the dissonance occurring between the temporal framework of a healthy and able-bodied person (myself, the researcher) and one who had a disease 'likely to cause rapid deterioration in their physical and mental capacities' coupled with 'a future that cannot be mapped out' (as Jackie, the Macmillan nurse, put it). Although for most people (such as myself), 'time is ordinarily experienced as a gearing towards the future' (Toombs 1995: 19; see also Gell 1992: 290), given this approach to time, it becomes obvious that, for patients with life-threatening illnesses, the future assumes an inherently problematic quality. Indeed, as Golander observes in her study of chronically ill geriatric patients:

> The arrow of time points ... to two courses of undesired change. One is related to further deterioration in health and the loss of those few remaining physical abilities still

under their control. The other entails the termination of life and the way by which death finds them.

(Golander 1995: 126)

Patients thus attempted to negotiate and resolve the problematic nature of the future by reordering and re-evaluating time: they downplayed the significance of forthcoming events (i.e. further deterioration, and ultimately their deaths) and focused upon past and present concerns. In most cases, the future was not denied or negated altogether; rather, it was displaced to the realm of a distant, abstract and hence non-threatening domain. Thus as one patient suggested, 'I try not to think, or worry, about what's likely to come next. I cope by taking one day at a time.' Patients often reinforced this type of remark by adding that they did not, at present, want to know any further details about their illness and the deterioration it was likely to cause. Their comments suggested that they were employing a conscious strategy to hold onto a 'normal' identity and sense of self in the present. Nettie, for example, originally developed breast cancer, and was admitted to day care after the cancer spread to the bones in her pelvis. After she had been attending day care for a couple of weeks, her hospital consultant told her that the cancer had also spread to her lungs. Inevitably, this meant that her life expectancy was likely to be comparatively short. Nevertheless, Nettie insisted that:

I try not to see myself as unwell at present. I really don't want to know what my cancer holds in store for me in the future. Yes, that would really scare me. I want to carry on living life normally for as long as I possibly can. I don't think that would be possible if I allowed myself to worry about what's waiting for me round the corner.

It was for this reason, as she went on to explain, that she had chosen not to discuss her latest diagnosis and its future implications with her family in any detail: 'If they know how serious my illness is now they'll stop treating me like I'm normal. They'll smother me and treat me like a child. I'm not ready for that yet.'

To some therapists (for example, the visitor from the hospice who I discuss later) patients such as Nettie could be seen as being in a state of 'denial'; an unrealistic position entailing serious psychic costs. My observations suggest, however, that the majority of day care patients were not in a state of denial as such. On the contrary, they appeared to exhibit what Gordon has described as 'contextual knowing', whereby, 'uncertainty is cultivated and manipulated socially and psychologically' by a patient as a strategy for holding onto their current identities, and thus remaining embedded within their existing social networks (1990: 283, 290). Indeed, Bluebond-Langner, in her study of leukaemic children, has noted that both the children and adults practised 'mutual pretence' because 'it offered each of them a way to fulfil the responsibilities necessary for maintaining membership in society, in the face of what threatened the fulfilment of social obligations and continued membership' (1978: 210). Examples such as these thus cast doubt upon Kübler-Ross' (1969) five-stage theory of dying, in which she suggests that patients move through a phase of denial and disbelief (followed by anger, bargaining and then depression) before finally reaching a stage of acceptance. Clearly, more complicated scenarios can, and do, occur in which patients do not simply switch between the stages identified by Kübler-Ross, but can express and experience such things as denial and acceptance simultaneously.

It was because patients had constructed – and attempted to live within – a present-orientated temporal framework that my reference to 'terminal illness' proved so problematic to Karen in the incident cited above. Clearly, it offended her subjective construction and experience of non-progressive time because the word 'terminal' connoted a projection into the future; a future, furthermore, which she associated with deterioration, decline and, ultimately, death.

A similar contradiction also often occurred between the temporal frameworks of patients and those of their families. Family members, in contrast to patients, were often keen to obtain as much information as possible about a patient's illness, and his or her likely prognosis, because they wanted to make plans for the future. On occasions when the temporal frameworks of the patient and carer became enmeshed, the conflict that ensued could be very severe. Fiona, for example, who had advanced cervical cancer, was extremely bitter after her husband had gone behind her back and researched her illness, thereby establishing that she probably had a prognosis of less than six months. Whilst Fiona was aware of the serious nature of her cancer, she had chosen not to 'dwell on it' or to discuss her prognosis in depth with her family, because she wanted her life to remain 'normal for as long as possible'.

Fiona's anxieties appeared to be well founded. Once her husband had completed his research, his behaviour altered markedly towards her. He changed their disabled daughter's attendance allowance into his own name without consulting her. When he did finally inform Fiona of his actions, he explained that he had to prepare for the future, a future in which she would be gone. Fiona complained that her husband had started treating her as if she were 'already dead'. She had always been the chief decision-maker in the family; now her husband was rapidly taking this role away from her.[7]

Fiona's problems escalated after her husband contacted her mother (then living abroad) to break the bad news to her. Her mother promptly flew over, installed herself in the couple's house, and took over the running of the household and the orchestration of Fiona's life. Fiona complained of 'feeling totally redundant, stifled and smothered' back at home. She pointed out that her mother even insisted on putting her into a wheelchair every time she wanted to go to the bathroom, in spite of the fact that she was well capable of walking there without assistance. Fiona, like Jane, felt she was being 'written off' by the stereotype of the 'dying person' which, in this instance, her family had projected onto her. In effect, the 'gap' Fiona was going to leave in her kinship network was already being filled before her death.

In the light of the above example, it is possible to understand why patients were sometimes so reluctant and unwilling for their families to have full knowledge of their prognosis. Yet the strategy of not sharing information could also have very detrimental effects. It was not uncommon for family members to suggest that they were so frustrated by a patient's unwillingness to talk about their illness and to make plans for the future, that they found they were withdrawing from the patient themselves. As one husband commented:

> I feel as if she's pulling away from me, and I know I'm pulling away from her. I can't get through to her anymore; it's so annoying because she doesn't want to talk about things. ... I get so frustrated that I've given up talking to her about anything.

The somewhat paradoxical situation that patients thus confronted was aptly summed up by the day care leader Kate, who suggested that, 'even those patients who have supportive families can still feel trapped within their families. Either they feel unable to talk openly about their illness, or, if they do, they feel that their family cannot understand them.'

When the above observations are considered together, it could be suggested that patients experienced a debasement of self and a loss of identity in several interrelated ways. Physical impairment made it difficult for patients to maintain social relationships and to perform tasks through which they felt themselves to be the agents of their own lives and the lives of others; physical signs of disease led to feelings of worthlessness and to negative responses from other people; also, patients and families became increasingly alienated and estranged from one another in terms of visions and plans relating to the future. As a consequence, many patients became dislodged from their networks of interpersonal relationships; this situation led them to experience a form of 'social death', wherein they had ceased to be 'active agent[s] in others' lives' (Mulkay 1993: 33).[8] Paradoxically then, as we shall see, one of the key factors which enabled patients to 'feel normal' and to 'return to a normal life' within the very 'un-normal' context of day care, was the opportunities it afforded patients to form 'pseudo-kinship' relationships with other members of the group.

Physical dependency

As important as these issues are, it was clear that feelings of despondency and low self-esteem were most commonly experienced by patients who found themselves, as a result of the debilitative impact of their illness, physically dependent upon others. Patients who suffered from poor mobility frequently expressed considerable anxiety that they had become a 'burden' to their family and friends – a phenomenon which is examined further in Chapter 3. Patients' feelings of low self-worth also became evident in the suggestion made by some that they had originally agreed to be admitted to day care more for their family's benefit than their own.[9] As Helen put it:

> I originally decided to come here for my husband. He had to give up his job to care for me. I know he gets sick of being stuck in the house with me all the time. ... Sometimes I feel really guilty because I know I've taken his life away from him. It's not fair on him, but neither of us really have a choice at the end of the day. ... At least this way he

gets one day a week where he can go out and do his own thing.

My interviews with patients' carers confirmed that their anxieties about the impact of their physically dependent state were often well founded. Members of the patients' family frequently expressed a high degree of ambivalence about taking on the role of carer since, in many respects, the difficulties they encountered were very similar to those of the patient: a sense of isolation and a change of self. This situation was highlighted very aptly by the widow of a former day care patient, who recounted her experience of being a carer in the following way:

> Families can't always help each other because they're too close. Families do get tired of it. I never resented my husband, but it did get to the stage where *I felt stripped bare inside*. Day care became his safety valve and mine. ... When my husband came to day care I got a whole day in which I could plan and do my own thing ... one day to look forward to, *one day to be free*.
>
> (widow, emphasis added)

I shall consider the complex effects of patients' illness and impairment upon the network of people involved with their care in the following chapter; for the moment I will concentrate upon the ways in which patients' loss of bodily autonomy, and thus their unreciprocated dependence upon others, led to a debasement of their personhood. Such a phenomenon has been recognised by Hockey and James who argue that the association of physical dependency with a loss of personhood stems directly from the contemporary 'Western' conception of the person as an autonomous and independent entity (1993: 107). Consequently, 'if the pursuit of individual freedom is the hallmark of personhood then all those unable, through dependency, to hold to this aim are cast in less than fully social roles' (ibid.).[10] As we shall see later, one of the ways in which a patient's status as a person was successfully reinstated within day care was through various informal strategies employed to mask, negotiate and redefine the hierarchical relationship between the 'dependent' patient and the staff and volunteers who provided his or her care.

As I examine below, all such strategies employed within the day care setting were, in many respects, in direct opposition to the formal model of the service. Whilst the latter was concerned with rehabilitating the patient through the provision and implementation of individualised packages of therapeutic care, the informal model of care (i.e. the 'alternative reality') became a site and framework for acts of collective solidarity and communalism.

Day care: a space for sustaining the self

I can laugh in day care, but I hurt when I'm back at home.
(Sara, patient)

This comment was proffered by Sara, the author of the poem at the start of this chapter, whilst she was chatting with some of the other patients. What it highlights is the disparity between her 'performance of self' (Goffman 1959) within day care, and her sense of self outside this setting. In day care, Sara was a cheerful and engaging patient who laughed and joked a lot with the other patients. However, she confided that back in her own home her feelings and behaviour were often very different: she frequently felt 'very angry, scared and alone'. Hence, day care had become her 'safe retreat'.

In the following sections I examine how, within day care, patients were able to 'feel normal' and to lead 'normal lives', which, as illustrated above, contrasted substantially with their experiences outside the day care setting. In arguing that patients exhibited one type of self (a 'normal' self) within day care and another seemingly contradictory self back in 'the community' (a 'diminished' self), I follow Butler's assertion that self-identity is an existential 'cultural performance', and thus a contextually dependent and variable effect 'of institutions, practices, discourses and multiple and diffuse points of origin' (1990: viii). Hence, as Ewing has similarly suggested, 'Western' (and other) persons can, and do, enact multiple, seemingly inconsistent 'self representations', which are context-dependent, and change when the context changes (1990: 251, 253).[11] The arguments of both writers thus concur closely with Schutz's idea of the existence of multiple realities, each characterised by its own 'finite province of meaning' (1967: 230), and its own peculiar cognitive style involving a specific time perspective, a specific form of self experience, and a specific form of sociality (1967: 232). The paradox then, as the work of these authors would seem to suggest, is that the 'Western' sense of interiorised selfhood is dependent upon it being reflected and confirmed by others (see p. 5).

The setting

As I noted in Chapter 1, day care was located in borrowed premises for the duration of the two-year pilot project. After the pilot project had been running for about six months, the Friends (see p. 20), in collaboration with the Cancer Relief Macmillan Fund, launched a major appeal to raise one million pounds from the local community. The appeal was set up to finance the construction of an extension to the hospice, so that day care could be housed in permanent purpose-built premises.[12] The new building would also accommodate a Resource Centre and additional teaching and office facilities. The appeal was extremely successful and the building was completed shortly after the pilot came to an end.

In spite of the temporary nature of the day care pilot, various 'stage props' (Goffman 1959: 32) were purchased to give the setting a 'homelike' appearance. These included items such as rugs, lamps, wall hangings, cushions, plants and floral crockery. The planned resemblance between day care and a home was even more apparent in the new purpose-built facility. This contained a fitted kitchen; a conservatory with patio; an activities room and a large day room furnished with easy chairs, settees, fitted carpets, a large fireplace and a Welsh-dresser displaying decorated plates. Day care was not unique in this respect because it is a common practice to design therapeutic environments so that they appear 'homelike'. As Godkin has observed, planners of therapeutic and rehabilitative services believe that, 'feelings of fear and isolation … are exacerbated by traditional care facilities which, in essence, remove a person physically from the familiarity of his [*sic*] regular surroundings' (1980: 82). McCourt Perring has similarly noted that social policy makers believe that 'settings constructed as "the community" or "family-like" ' (1994: 168) enable client groups to 'be more independent and more integrated socially' (ibid.).

The impact of space and environment upon behaviour has now been extensively theorised within the anthropological, sociological and social geographical literature. Buttimer, for example, observes that buildings and architectural spaces are designed to shape and reflect the interactions taking place within them (1980: 24). Ardener similarly notes that once space has been bounded and shaped it is no longer a neutral background; it exerts its own influence (1981:

12). However, as Ardener further suggests, whilst space can define action, 'the presence of individuals in space in turn determines its nature' (1981: 12–13), since space also has a 'lived', 'subjective component' (Buttimer 1980: 24; see also Ingold 1995). The latter observation held particularly true for day care: whilst the day care 'theatre of action' (Ardener 1981: 12) was designed to foster a therapeutic and rehabilitative ethos, it was accorded and imbued with a very different meaning by its participants. It is thus to the day-to-day activities occurring within day care that I now turn.

The routine

The day care routine remained fairly stable on a day-to-day and a week-to-week basis. A typical day began at 9.00 a.m. for staff and volunteers. As the pilot project was located in borrowed premises, a large amount of behind-the-scenes work was necessary to prepare the room for the patients' arrival. The volunteers were responsible for setting up the room, which involved laying out the patterned rugs, hanging pictures and tapestries on the walls, arranging the easy chairs in a large circle, and placing plants and flowers (flower arrangements were regularly donated by a local women's voluntary group) in various parts of the room. A relaxation tape or popular classical music was put on to play just before the patients were due to arrive.

Patients started arriving at 10.00 a.m. Some were dropped off by family and friends, but the majority were brought in by volunteer drivers who had special training in lifting and handling. Patients were greeted by the staff and volunteers and invited to take a seat in the circular arrangement of chairs; those with poor mobility, and those in wheelchairs, were given physical assistance by staff and volunteers. Volunteers offered and served hot drinks and biscuits to patients. Family members and volunteer drivers were also invited to stay for coffee, although few took up this offer in practice. Most patients reached day care by 10.30, although some occasionally arrived later if their weakness and lethargy was such that they found it difficult to get out of bed too early.

All members of the group interacted informally with one another over morning coffee. Staff and volunteers interspersed themselves with patients, which led visitors to comment that they had difficulties identifying who the patients actually were – a situation which also stemmed from the fact that all participants usually dressed casually, and staff and volunteers were often of similar ages to patients. Whilst some patients used this first part of the morning to query matters such as their diet and medication, the bulk of interactions occurring amongst patients, and between patients, staff and volunteers, took the form of what Jerrome has termed 'small frame conversations' (1992: 83). Conversations of this type, as Jerrome suggests, serve to provide 'a mosaic of non-critical listening and talking which meets the need for self-expression and the reassurance of worth' (ibid.). Staff, volunteers and patients alike would reminisce and share anecdotes about family and friends. It was also common for patients and volunteers to bring in photos of events such as family gatherings, holidays and weddings to share with the whole group.[13]

After morning coffee, Kate, the occupational therapist, encouraged patients to move into a separate room and participate in therapeutic activities such as painting, making tapestries and constructing bird and jewellery boxes. In practice, however, most patients opted to remain seated with one another in the main room and to continue with their conversations.[14]

The participants congregated back in the main room at approximately midday for drinks (again served by the volunteers) followed by a light sandwich lunch.[15] All members of the group – including staff and volunteers – sat together at the same table for this meal. At lunch time, it was particularly common for patients, staff and volunteers alike to spontaneously refer to the group as 'one big family'. The significance of the use of this 'family' metaphor will be examined later. After lunch, patients reassembled in the circle of chairs for a relaxation session, which the two staff members took turns to conduct. The volunteers would also normally participate in these sessions, provided they had finished tidying and washing up after lunch. Some patients slept after the relaxation sessions, while others continued with their conversations, participated in communal card games, or received individual massages from Lucy, the day care nurse.

Afternoon tea was served at 3.00 and followed a similar group format to morning coffee. Soon afterwards, volunteer drivers and family members arrived to take patients home. The volunteers then proceeded to restore the room to its former condition and return the various 'stage props' to the cupboard.

Patients appeared to attach considerable importance to the day care routine, which, as already indicated, remained fairly consistent from one week to the next. Indeed they could become quite distressed if an element in the routine was changed, such as on the odd occasion when the relaxation session was omitted. I also noticed that some patients felt it important to sit in the same chair in the same location every week. A couple of times during my fieldwork an outing to a local pub was substituted for the sandwich lunch, although excursions of this kind were rarely planned well in advance, since staff were only able to accurately gauge patients' physical and mental conditions on their arrival. The occupational therapist, Kate, also occasionally organised entertainment in day care, such as afternoon concerts. Nevertheless, communal activities of this type were slotted into the established routine, rather than compromising or over-riding the existing format.[16]

It seemed, then, that a rather stable routine had developed in day care because it served to provide a locus of continuity in patients' lives – lives, which as highlighted above, were otherwise characterised by loss and deterioration. A similar observation has been developed by Hazan in his study of a day centre for elderly Jewish people in London. Hazan points to the 'repetitive' nature of most activities taking place within 'the Centre', which, he argues, led to a stifling of 'innovation and creativity' (1980: 143; 1984). This phenomenon, he suggests, served to bring about a 'freezing' of the participants' social conditions, which, in reality, was incongruous with 'their actual experience of accelerating deterioration' (1980: 89). The social construction of time within day care will be examined further below.

Constructing an 'alternative reality': patients as actors

> Little of what we do here now stemmed from conscious decision ... we ... responded to the patients.
>
> (Lucy, day care nurse)

> I'm the same Pauline here as I am with my family and friends. It's what the patients want and expect. If we volunteers were to be any different, day care just wouldn't work.
>
> (Pauline, volunteer)

The above ethnographic account begins to highlight the difference that had evolved between the individualised, formal rehabilitative model of day care and the informal communal-based practices which actually occurred within the setting. This is not a unique phenomenon: Wright, in her anthropological study of bureaucratic organisations, has noted that a contradiction often develops between formal organisational structures, and the informal ways in which individuals and groups within the organisation actually relate to one another (1994: 17). Furthermore, as the statements above suggest, patients were actively involved in the deconstruction and subsequent reconstruction of the day care environment. As those working there said repeatedly, 'we responded to the patients'; 'it's what the patients want and expect'. Hence, it seems reasonable to argue that the informal model of care developed as it did because it was more directly in line with what the patients actually needed and wanted.[17]

Since the 1980s, anthropological and sociological theory has paid substantial attention to the concepts of social agency, praxis, and the performative nature of embodied action (Ortner 1984; Crossley 1995; Shilling 1991). Whilst practice-orientated approaches recognise the impact of social structures upon human action, social structures are also regarded as the outcome of the 'transformative capacity' (Giddens 1984: 15) of human agents/actors. Thus, as Moore suggests:

> Shifts in meaning can result from a reordering of practical activities. If meaning is given to the organization of space through practice, it follows that small changes in procedure can provide new interpretations of spatial layouts. Such layouts provide potential commentaries on established ways of doing things and divisions of privilege. Shifting the grounds of meaning, reading against the grain, is often something done through practice, that is, through day-to-day activities which take place in symbolically structured space.
>
> (Moore 1994: 83)

Practice theory, furthermore, recognises that 'systems' are not necessarily harmonious integrated wholes (Ortner 1984: 148). Changes from within a system can thus come about as a result of actors 'experiencing the complexities of their situations and attempting to solve the problems posed by those situations' (1984: 151). In the case of day care, it would appear that patients encountered a contradiction between the formal model of care with its strong rehabilitative focus, and their actual subjective need for an integrated, on-going system of interpersonal, psycho-social support. Hence the emergence of an 'alternative reality' which diverged from the formal objectives of the service. Ortner, however, has also developed the Weberian perspective that major, long-term social change 'does not for the most part come about as an *intended* consequence of action. Change is largely a by-product, an *un*intended consequence of action, however rational action may have been' (1984: 157, original emphasis). Thus, 'society' and 'history' are 'rarely the products the actors themselves set out to make' (ibid., see also Giddens 1984). This observation will be shown to be particularly pertinent in the final section of this chapter, where I discuss the impact of the evaluation on the long-term future of the day care service.

The central performative role adopted by patients in the creation of day care's 'alternative reality' became apparent even on my first day of fieldwork. After the staff had introduced me to the patients and explained the nature of my research interests and involvement with the evaluation to them, I was happy to sit quietly at the periphery of the group and make some initial observations. However, I was quickly taken to task by one patient, Rose, who chided me in the following way: 'Julia, if you want to become one of us, you're going to have to learn to join in.' Both aspects of Rose's comment, 'becoming one of us' and 'joining in', proved central to the ways in which the staff, volunteers and I were drawn into interactions and relationships with patients.

As my account of the day care routine indicates, all participants – patients, staff and volunteers – interacted with one another as a communal group. This communal group ethos was especially apparent in the acts of commensality which occurred several times during each day. The whole group sat together for morning coffee and afternoon tea, and shared a communal meal at the same table. This practice had not been planned when the pilot project was first set up; when I interviewed the two members of staff, they told me that they had originally tried to take their lunch break separately from patients. Similarly, it had originally been planned that the volunteers would have their own break after they had served lunch to the patients and cleared and tidied up. However, staff and volunteers quickly came to recognise how much the patients expected and valued their presence, hence they stopped eating separately from them.

The importance that day care patients clearly attached to regular commensal rituals can be understood in terms of their role in breaking down the hierarchical distinctions between the 'carers' (staff and volunteers) and the 'cared for' (patients). It is almost certainly no coincidence that the staff and volunteers not only interspersed themselves with patients, but also consumed the same food and drink.[18] An egalitarian ethic was also apparent in a number of other informal practices which took place in the day-to-day setting. An unspoken policy had developed, for example, whereby staff, volunteers and patients addressed one another on a strictly first-name basis; the emphasis being on treating each member as a person in their own right, as Strathern's study of modern English kin terms suggests (1992b: 19–20). Such behaviour stands in contrast to the patterns occurring within other institutions such as hospitals and residential homes. Hockey and James have observed that in these settings staff often engage in 'pet naming' and other infantilising practices, which, they suggest, serve to reinforce a negative status amongst elderly and disabled client groups (1993: 10).

In a similar and related vein, staff and volunteers had adopted an informal code in which they dressed in the same ways as patients. Again, this behaviour pitted them in contrast to professionals working in other medical settings. Lawler has observed that one of the reasons why medical staff normally wear uniforms is because uniforms serve to create a boundary between the professional carer and patient (1991: 152); an argument which ties in with Foucault's observation that medical professionals remain 'at a distance' from their patients (1993: 136). Whilst the former constitute the 'knowing subjects', the latter become the 'objects' of the medical 'gaze' (1993: 137). This type of distancing strategy was clearly absent from day care; indeed, when I questioned one of the volunteers about why she chose to wear casual clothes she offered the following remark: 'I suppose it's because the patients don't usually feel well enough to dress up themselves.' The two members of staff also recognised that they broke down their professional barriers – and thus the differences between themselves and the patients – by wearing their own clothes. When one of the patients asked Kate, the occupational therapist, why she did not wear a uniform she offered the following comment: 'We don't hide behind our uniforms here, we are what we are.'

Brotchie and Hills have noted that receiving care can be both degrading and humiliating for patients, and thus leads to a debasement of their personhood (1991: 9). Yet it appears that various strategies had emerged within day care which subsumed and negated the differences between the carers (the staff and volunteers) and patients, thereby helping, I would suggest, to make the dependency status of the latter less apparent.

Deconstructing and reconstructing concepts of care

The day care 'alternative reality' was constructed and sustained through a number of other related, dependent processes. One of the most important of these concerned the ways in which the idea of 'care' as an emotional, structural and ideological force was appropriated and redefined by patients and staff in their day-to-day interactions, and actively used in the negotiation of social reality (Lutz and White 1986: 420).

The work of various feminist scholars has highlighted the multi-dimensional meanings encompassed within 'care' and 'carework'. Ungerson (1987) and Dalley (1988), for example, differentiate 'care' into its 'caring for' and 'caring about' components: 'The first is to do with the tasks of tending another person, the second with feelings for another person' (Dalley 1988: 8). Graham makes a similar distinction when she refers to caring as both 'taking charge' and as 'feeling concern'; as 'labour' and as 'love' (1983: 13; see also Lewis 1986). James, likewise, divides carework into physical labour, emotional labour and its organisational components (1992). Most studies have focused upon the reproduction of the contemporary stereotypical 'Western' family where it is argued that the emotional and physical components of care are inseparable (Graham 1991; Dalley 1988: 8). Thus, as La Fontaine has observed, whilst an imbalance of power exists between 'independent' adults and 'dependent' children (1990: 77), family relationships also find their expression in egalitarian notions of sharing, altruism and 'natural affection' (1990: 152).

In contrast, however, Thomas has observed that, where care is conceived as occurring separately from the reproduction of the family, it is defined more heavily in terms of 'tending' to 'dependants' (1993). Hence, relationships between professional carers and patients tend to be particularly hierarchical and unequal, with the former 'taking charge' (Hugman 1994: 10). James explains the differences between institutional and family practices of care as stemming in part from the fact that, in institutional settings, staff regard physical labour as much more tangible and readily identifiable than its emotional counterpart (1992: 496). Further-more, physical tasks 'also have an additional meaning since they

are the principal component of "work" in the sense of paid labour'
(ibid.).

The hierarchical nature of care, characteristic of an institutional
setting, was indeed evident in day care's Operational Policy, where
the roles of staff and volunteers were defined primarily in terms of
their physical aspects, namely, 'tending to' and 'caring for' patients.
Hence, as I have already described in Chapter 1, heavy emphasis
was given in the staff's and volunteers' job descriptions to practical
chores and to providing patients with physical assistance, such as
helping disabled patients to the bathroom. As I have begun to
highlight above, however, the physical components of care enacted
by staff and volunteers were, in practice, superseded by the more
altruistic concern of 'caring about' patients. Such a shift in
emphasis was particularly evident in the informal ways in which
volunteers constructed and perceived their roles. When I invited
them to reflect upon their work in day care, all acknowledged the
importance of their 'housekeeping' chores (e.g. washing and tidying
up), but the majority, nevertheless, suggested these duties were of
secondary importance to offering 'friendship' and 'tender loving
care' to patients. As Olive suggested:

> it's caring that's really important; treating the patients like
> people and not just as their cancer. I feel really bonded to
> them. They're like friends, like family, I suppose.

Another volunteer, Kathy, commented:

> I like coming here and making friends with the patients.
> They're not in the least bit self-centred. It's nice that they
> want to know what you've been doing too. ... I grow really
> fond of them.

Similarly, when the two staff members talked informally about
their work in day care the following remark arose:

> The patients here are very special. They have a lot of
> warmth and love to give as well as to receive. People come
> here to be loved and cared for. It's being able to offer this
> that makes our work so rewarding.

The staff's and volunteers' perception of their roles was reflected
and reinforced in the patients' expectations of the service. In their

day-to-day conversations, patients frequently commented upon why they found coming to day care so helpful:

> Feeling cared for and knowing someone wants to listen. ... It's very traumatic to feel so ill ... you're badly hurt physically and emotionally and you need someone to care.
>
> (Sarah)

> It's the love and companionship I like; it's so good to talk and feel I still matter.
>
> (Margaret)

> Company ... having someone to listen and care. ... We're all kindred spirits. We all look out for each other here.
>
> (Jan)

> It's all the love and friendliness we can offer each other. I'd feel totally lost if I had to stop coming.
>
> (Mark)

The frequent references made by patients, staff and volunteers alike to the emotional elements of care is in itself highly significant. Lutz, in her seminal study *Unnatural Emotions* (1988), has challenged the idea that emotions are 'natural', 'pre-cultural' and 'innate'. Rather, she argues that emotions should be understood as an index of social relationships; as an emergent product of social life:

> the use of emotion concepts, as elements of ideological practice, involves negotiation over the meaning of events, over rights and morality, over control of resources ... over the entire range of issues that concern human groups. ... Once de-essentialized, emotion can be viewed as a cultural and interpersonal process of naming, justifying and persuading by people in relationship to each other.
>
> (Lutz 1988: 5)

Thus emotion words are not simply passive reflections of social reality; they are actively employed 'to negotiate aspects of social reality and to create that reality' (Lutz 1988: 10). A similar argument is made by Medick and Sabean who point to the role of emotions as a 'grammar', or symbolic system, embedded in social relationships (1984: 3).

Once emotions are recognised as socially constituted expressions and determinants of experience and practice it becomes possible to understand why words such as 'love', 'friendship', 'caring' and 'kindred spirits' were employed so widely and publicly in the day care setting. As I have already indicated, staff, volunteers and patients were in a potentially strained relationship with one another, since patients constituted a physically 'dependent' group, whereas staff and volunteers comprised a group upon whom they relied for assistance with physical and practical matters. It could be argued, therefore, that the use of emotion concepts served on one level as a strategy for mediating and negotiating the potentially unequal relationship between 'carers' and 'cared for', by enabling the hierarchical (i.e. the physical) components of care to be masked and overridden by its more altruistic, emotional aspects. Indeed, the enactment and expression of emotions provided the one means by which patients were able to place themselves on an equal footing with staff and volunteers, precisely because emotions were the one aspect of care which they were actually able to *reciprocate*. As the quotes above indicate, patients 'looked out for' staff and volunteers and took an active interest in hearing anecdotes about their families and hobbies. I should emphasise that I am not suggesting that emotions did not exist as genuine – and genuinely felt – experiences within day care. Rather I am attempting to understand why emotions and emotion words were expressed so publicly and with such high frequency by day care participants.

In light of the above analysis, it also becomes possible to understand why the 'family' metaphor was employed so regularly by patients, staff and volunteers alike in their day-to-day interactions. One obvious explanation for this practice is that the word 'family' aptly embodied and gave expression to the types of interpersonal relationships which were formed within the group. As I indicated earlier, many patients admitted to the service were suffering from social isolation and valued day care as a type of 'surrogate family' in which they could forge close personal ties with one another, and thereby preserve the exterior components of their selves (see Chapter 5). The use of the term 'family' may also have helped to 'personalise' day care, making it seem less like a formal institution. Yet, as La Fontaine has argued, 'like many other key cultural values in other societies, "the family" contains multiple ambiguities, even contradictions, within the whole complex of notions it represents' (1990: 184). As I pointed out above, one of the key ambiguities La Fontaine identifies is that 'the family' simultaneously conveys notions of power and inequality on the one hand and altruism and equality on the other. This double-sided nature of 'the family' metaphor, it could be argued, enabled it to act as a particularly powerful medium for contesting, masking and re-negotiating the dependency relationships occurring between patients, staff and volunteers. A further ambiguity in the concept is suggested by Graham's observation that the day-to-day work occurring within families meets the needs of *able-bodied* adults as well as children and other persons with dependency needs (Graham 1991). Indeed, it is no coincidence that day care patients used non-hierarchical kinship terms such as 'kindred spirits' when referring to one another and to staff and volunteers. As Hockey and James have suggested, 'relations of equality can be created among groups and individuals otherwise structurally set apart from one another, through the metaphoric use of collateral kinship terminology such as "sister", "brother" or "cousin" ' (1993: 118), whereas descent terminology (e.g. 'mother', 'father') is constitutive of relationships of dependency and inequality (ibid.).

Several further, related strategies were also employed within day care to break down the identities of the patients as the 'objects' and 'recipients' of 'care'. Consider, for example, the following exchanges which occurred when a staff member or volunteer 'tended' directly to a 'dependent' patient:

PATTY (PATIENT):   I feel really pampered here.
JUDY (VOLUNTEER): Well you're *special*.
(extract from a conversation whilst Judy was serving Patty a pre-lunch drink; emphasis added)

BEATRICE (PATIENT):   Oh you do spoil me here.
LUCY (NURSE):   Well you *deserve* it.
(extract from a conversation whilst Lucy was helping Beatrice with her tapestry; emphasis added)

What is evident in these interactions is the attempt by both parties to transpose the identity of the patient from that of a 'dependant' to someone seen as 'deserving' and/or 'special'. This process, I suggest, made it possible for patients to receive care as a 'right' or an 'entitlement' rather than due to the more demoralising and degrading reason of 'need'.

Patients' experiences of 'dependency' were also, to some extent, mitigated and overridden by the present-bound, non-linear temporal framework that had been constructed within day care (see below). As Mauss has argued in *The Gift* (1990), the giving of objects and services normally creates a hierarchical relationship of indebtedness between the 'donor' and 'recipient', until the 'debt' has been discharged at some future stage in time. Within day care, however, the concept of the future was negated and underplayed by all participants. It could be argued, therefore, that the emphasis given to present-orientated concerns afforded a secondary gain in that it enabled patients to receive physical care without entailing a sense of indebtedness and therefore of dependency. In this respect, day care echoed patterns observed in anthropological studies of egalitarian societies and sects. In these social groups, as Golander has noted, relationships of equality are reflected and reinforced through the construction of cyclical, non-progressive time (1995: 132).

Day care: a space for masking deterioration and dependency

When the above observations are considered together, it is apparent that what was being constructed within day care was an acceptable means by which staff and volunteers could 'tend to' and 'care for' patients without the dependency status of the latter being reinforced. This interactional model thus made it possible for 'carers' to 'take over' and perform tasks for patients (e.g. fetching items which they required) without patients necessarily experiencing a debasement of self.

Another significant consequence of this model of care was, I suggest, that it enabled patients to remain static within space, thus masking from themselves and others the often rapid bodily decline that occurred over the period they were attending day care. It is no coincidence that when day care moved into its new, purpose-built premises (which were substantially larger than those housing the pilot project), volunteers frequently commented that they found their work considerably more physically demanding. In the act of tending to patients and performing tasks on their behalf, it was the volunteers who did all the moving through space; in the new premises, the volunteers had considerably more space to negotiate and move around in.

Other spatial and temporal strategies were also employed within day care to mask patients' bodily deterioration. It is, for example, salient that the whole group normally sat together in a circular arrangement of chairs. This seating layout enabled the whole group to converse and interact with one another without individual patients actually having to attempt to move around. It is also significant that the types of craft activity made available within day care were those which required minimal physical strength on the part of patients, the most obvious being stencilling and tapestry-making kits. The occupational therapist, Kate, also made a point of buying expensive kits, so that she could be sure that the end-products would always look professional, rather than amateurish and childish.

The time conspiracy: the negation of future-orientated time and the 'denial' of death

As I indicated earlier, the concepts of the future and future-orientated time presented particular difficulties to day care patients because, for them, it was associated with their physical decline and a consequent loss of self. To maintain day care as a 'safe haven' it was therefore necessary for all involved to participate in practices which served to distance patients from their futures and, in particular, the physical reality of deterioration and death. As I now examine, a number of strategies were employed by participants to deconstruct and re-order day care's temporal events, thereby enabling directional progressive time to be displaced, to some extent, by a present-bound perspective. In suggesting that the temporal framework within day care could be reconstructed, I am building upon the arguments made by anthropologists such as Munn, Hazan and Gell that time is a culturally variable and hence a socially manipulable resource (Munn 1992; Hazan 1980, 1984; Gell 1992).

It is no coincidence that whilst patients frequently reminisced and shared anecdotes about their pasts within the day care setting, it was extremely rare for them to discuss events extending beyond their immediate futures with one another.[19] The future, both as a concept and as a topic of conversation within the group, became taboo, particularly in instances where it could be associated with the anticipated deterioration and death of individual members. This phenomenon is made particularly evident in the following ethnographic vignettes.

On one occasion, a new female patient who used to work as an astrologer brought her computer into day care so she could do the other patients' astrological charts. All the patients declined to have their futures read. On that particular day, in fact, they were only too happy to move into another room and participate in therapeutic activities, leaving the woman sitting alone in the main room. The incident was not discussed by the other patients, and the woman did not bring her computer in again.

The staff also informed me that, when day care was first opened, the hospice counsellor used to make regular visits. This counsellor held particularly strong views about how day care should operate. When I interviewed her, she suggested that patients should be encouraged to talk openly and frankly about the incurable nature of their illness, so that they could make the necessary practical and emotional preparations for their forthcoming deaths.[20] Her opinion, however, was clearly not shared by patients. A wave of tension used to hit the room as soon as she entered the day care premises. The counsellor stopped making visits after it became apparent that patients were doing everything possible to avoid talking to her.

Patients with unrealistic expectations regarding the future were also ostracised by other members of the group. One notable incident occurred when day care was visited by a 50-year-old man who had just been informed by his doctors that his cancer of the prostate could not be cured. His Macmillan nurse encouraged him to go and see the set-up in day care, so that he could decide whether he wanted to attend on a regular basis. In a conversation with the staff and other patients, this man expressed particularly strong views about what his long-term expectations of the service would be. He proposed setting up a committee with other patients to plan trips to locations such as Boulogne and the theatres in London. Most patients sat in a stunned and bemused silence, though one did curtly point out that she didn't think most of them would be capable of participating in such ambitious ventures. The visitor left very abruptly, aware that he had not received a particularly warm reception from the other patients. As soon as he had departed, he became the brunt of their jokes, with patients expressing relief that he would probably not return.

Evidently, patients were instrumental in constructing and sustaining a present-bound temporal framework within day care, into which the past could also be incorporated (e.g. through showing old photographs) to construct an 'autobiography of self' which was free from the painful constraints of their current state of atrophied personhood. It became very clear to me that patients embraced experiences from the past with as much strength and vigour as they rejected and distanced themselves from topics alluding to the future. Indeed, one of the most popular events organised within day care required patients to reminisce extensively. In the event concerned, members of the English Touring Opera were invited by the day care leader to put on an afternoon concert. These musicians produced a very imaginative and innovative performance in which patients, staff and volunteers were invited to share their memories of childhood holidays. Every patient participated willingly in this venture, and the various topics and themes emerging from their anecdotes were incorporated by one of the musicians into the lines and verses of a song, whilst another wrote a simple tune to accompany the words. All the participants sang along to the final composition and the main chorus was repeated several times on the patients' request. Patients enthused about this particular concert for weeks and even months later.

Whilst the construction of the day care 'alternative reality' was clearly very dependent upon the mediation and control of events taking place within its immediate confines, it was also strongly reliant upon the maintenance of the setting as a physically and symbolically bounded entity. It was in this regard that staff and volunteers played a particularly instrumental role: they responded sympathetically and sensitively to patients' feelings and needs by mediating and filtering various potentially threatening events that occurred at day care's fringes. For instance, the day care pilot was located in a building situated mid-way between the hospice and the mortuary. This meant that after a hospice patient died, the porters had to wheel the corpse (contained in a casket) directly past day care's premises. This practice caused considerable antagonism between day care staff and porters, particularly on occasions in the summer when patients were sitting outside the day care building. If a porter was seen moving a body, one of the staff members or volunteers would send him back to the hospice, and instruct him to move the corpse after all the patients had gone home. When day care moved into its new premises, attached directly to the hospice, the following memo was sent out:

> Now the new Centre has opened, day care patients are able to see patients being removed to the mortuary by the porter. Therefore if within day care hours, please telephone the day centre and ask them to close the blinds. Where

possible patients [i.e. hospice patients who had recently died] may stay in the viewing room until out of hours.

Staff also employed various symbolic and metaphoric strategies to distance patients from the news of the deterioration of other members of their group. When a patient became too unwell to attend day care, staff would offer explanatory phrases such as 'she's feeling a little more poorly today' or 'he's not feeling his usual self at the moment' to soften the reality of that patient's decline. In contrast, behind the scenes comments such as 'she's going down fast' or 'he's dying' would be proffered in a briefing session with the volunteers before patients actually arrived. However, when the news reached the day care staff that a former patient had died (often patients did not die until several weeks or months after their final visit), staff did share this information with patients. Nevertheless, the news of a patient's death was disclosed and managed in such a way as to minimise damage to the day care 'alternative reality'. For instance, one of the volunteers informed me that the staff had originally planned to light a candle when a patient died, and to allocate time so that the whole group could reminisce together about the deceased person. This communal ritual did not occur once during my fieldwork, in spite of the fact that twelve patients died during that period. Instead, an alternative practice had emerged. Patients were taken to one side by staff and individually informed of the news of another member's death. On a couple of occasions, a bereavement counsellor was brought in and individual patients who had grown particularly close to the deceased person were offered the opportunity to discuss the death privately in a separate room. The staff justified this new practice on the basis that the deceased person was generally not known to all members of the group. Consequently, they suggested that it was unnecessary and unfair to bring up the topic of death in front of patients who were not personally affected by the news. Yet, it is also evident that this practice served to keep the topic of death at the fringes of the group; a practice, furthermore, that appeared to be embraced by most patients. On several occasions during my fieldwork, patients actually claimed they did not remember the former group member when the news of his or her death was broken to them. The patient's death was thus quickly glossed over and bypassed.

The earlier discussion of 'contextual knowing' is, I suggest, helpful in understanding why these various strategies were enacted to downplay future-orientated time, and its association with deterioration and death. I did not get the impression that day care patients, as a general rule, were actually in a state of denial about death; indeed, when I interviewed patients in private several informed me that when back in their own homes, they often read the obituary column in their local newspaper. Rather, it appears that patients, staff and volunteers jointly conspired in keeping deterioration and death 'at a distance' within day care because this practice was necessary to enable it to be sustained as a 'living' space.

It is, nevertheless, important to recognise that the creation of the day care 'safe haven' was, by its very nature, a fragile and tenuous process. Consequently, incidents did occasionally occur when the 'alternative reality' was undermined by the very existence of the suffering, deterioration and death that it sought to mask and negate.

Shortly before I started my fieldwork, three members of the 'Thursday group' had died in quick succession. It was very unusual for so many deaths to occur within such a short period, and this made it extremely difficult for the topic of death to be kept at the periphery of the group. Morale amongst the three remaining patients became extremely low. One woman, Beth, began talking repeatedly of her own anxieties about dying, apparently reducing the other two patients to tears. Both of these patients became so distressed that they asked to be discharged, leaving Beth as the sole attendee. This situation led Beth to also request a discharge. None of the patients asked to be readmitted at a later date.

On another occasion, the 'Friday group' fragmented after one of its former members, Tom, came back unexpectedly after being absent for six weeks. Tom was 40 and had cancer of the pancreas, which can be very aggressive in its later stages. The last time the others had seen him he had looked comparatively well, but by the time he returned, patients and staff alike had considerable difficulties recognising him. He had lost a substantial amount of weight and was suffering from mental confusion. He was also vomiting heavily and needed an enema. The staff speculated that Tom's wife had 'dumped' him with them, because she had reached a stage where she felt 'totally unable to cope at home'. They also expressed some anxiety that Tom might actually die in the day care premises. Tom's degree of deterioration was so severe that it could not be masked, and this visible degeneration had a significant impact upon all those present. Several patients were reduced to tears, and one woman was so upset that she requested an immediate appointment with her Macmillan nurse and told her she would not be coming to day care again. Another patient also stopped attending at this time, although she did not offer staff an explanation. When Kate later reflected upon this incident, she concluded that, 'it really wasn't fair to expose the patients so dramatically to what they can expect to happen to them at some stage in the future'.

Incidents of this type were, nevertheless, comparatively rare. Patients generally became too weak and lethargic to attend day care weeks, and sometimes even months, before their deaths occurred. Consequently, other patients were not normally exposed to the final stages of their deterioration. To a large extent, then, it was possible for a 'safe haven' to be sustained and reproduced. In fact, as I now go on to examine, the greatest challenge to day care stemmed somewhat ironically from its very success in providing 'a safe retreat' for patients.

The impact of the evaluation: conflict between 'rational' and 'emotional' concepts of care

As I indicated earlier, day care was established as a rehabilitative stepping stone to help patients adjust to the diagnosis of a life-threatening illness. As a consequence, it was anticipated by the NHS management and other planners of the service that it would be possible to discharge patients back into 'the community' once their eight weeks of care had finished. Patients, however, were often very reluctant to be discharged, since for them, day care constituted a 'safe retreat' from the outside world. Day care, as a consequence, became what could be termed a form of 'social morphine' for many of its patients. As Helen put it simply: 'Coming to day care is addictive. I'm so scared that they're going to try to discharge me. It would feel like I was being kicked out of the nest.' Tom (then at an early stage in his illness) similarly suggested that, 'I'd feel absolutely lost if I had to stop coming because of the support and having people who care. I'll be in more need of day care as the months go on and my disease progresses.'

The strong value patients attached to coming regularly to day care created a dilemma for the two members of staff. Both recognised that most patients were in need of an ongoing system of psycho-social support, particularly because the majority were only referred at a late stage in their illness, by which time they were often deteriorating quite rapidly.[21] Hence, as Kate suggested, many patients needed to attend day care indefinitely because they were 'having to make continual adjustments to changing circumstances'. In practice, therefore, day care's staff often covertly re-referred patients as soon as their care 'packages' had expired.[22] Kate explained her rationale in the following terms: 'It's not fair to discharge patients when they become very unwell. It would be like imposing yet another social death on them at a time when they're having to confront their actual deaths.'

The staff's informal practice of re-referring patients did not, however, become fully apparent to the NHS management until it was documented in the evaluation report. The statistical data laid out in the report revealed that over half the patients had been re-referred as soon as their eight-week care packages had come to an end,[23] and several had been attending the service continuously for more than a year. Following receipt of the evaluation, the Health Commission (the 'purchasers') backed down from its verbal commitment to fund the service once the pilot project came to an end. In a meeting set up with the NHS Trust (the 'providers') and the Friends to discuss the Health Commission's annual strategy for funding the region's palliative care services, their rationale became evident:

> What we have to consider is how many of our residents are going through and at what costs. The bottom line is that day care is not a cost-effective service, because so many patients are re-referred.
>
> (representative from the Health Commission)

As the representative from the Health Commission went on to explain, only limited finances were available for funding palliative care services and, consequently, 'the butter will have to be spread thinly on the bread to ensure the most equitable access to resources'. They could not, therefore, justify funding 'a Rolls Royce service that offers high quality care to a few but nothing to the rest'.[24]

Thus, as I indicated in Chapter 1, the evaluation constituted an arena in which day care's formal and informal models came into direct confrontation with one another for the first time. As a consequence, a latent conflict was brought to the surface; one which could be understood as the 'interlocked contradiction' (Hugman 1994: 1) occurring between the Health Commission's professional, 'rational', 'purchaser' concerns of cost-effectiveness and cost-accountability and day care's informal, 'emotional' constructions of care as altruistic and axiomatically ongoing (Roper 1994: 91; Webb 1985).

It is, indeed, highly pertinent that the Health Commission did not change its decision, in spite of the emotional appeals made in the meeting by representatives from the Friends and the Healthcare Trust to take the qualitative aspects of the report into consideration. I had contributed the bulk of this data. Extracts from my interviews with patients, their families, staff members and volunteers were used to highlight patients' experiences of suffering outside of day care, and thus to indicate the strong importance they attached to attending the service on a regular, long-term basis.[25] Upon reflecting on my own contribution to the evaluation, however, it is apparent that it actually had no bearing upon the final decision made by the Health Commission, particularly if one looks at broader cultural shifts and trends. As Kleinman and Kleinman have observed, contemporary Euro-American cultural rhetoric 'is changing from the language of caring to the language of efficiency and cost' (1996: 14). It is no coincidence that several representatives from the Health Commission confessed they had not even read the qualitative sections of the report; in their opinion, the qualitative data did not constitute an 'objective indicator' upon which 'rational choice' decisions concerning 'allocation of scarce resources' could be made (Kleinman and Kleinman 1996: 14).[26] One could argue that these members of the Health Commission held a very different view of reality to the staff and patients in day care; the Health Commission's reality was dominated by economic concerns (see Chapter 1).

In the introduction to an edition of *Daedalus* which is devoted to the topic of 'social suffering', the editors point to a 'moral dilemma' that stems from the gap between the 'representation' and 'responsibility' for suffering:

> What we represent and how we represent it prefigure what we will, or will not, do to intervene. What is not pictured is not real. Much of routinized misery is invisible; much that is made visible is not ordinary or routine.
>
> (Kleinman *et al.* 1996: xiii)

Hence, in the same volume, Kleinman and Kleinman warn of the dangers of 'configuring social suffering as an economic indicator'

(1996: 14) within models of health and social development. Such a practice, they suggest, denies that 'suffering is a social experience' (ibid.), with the implication that the suffering of individual people will not be successfully recognised or addressed within dominant cultural paradigms. This dilemma was recognised by the day care leader, Kate. When she heard the news that the Health Commission had not agreed to fund the service, she offered one cynical comment to me: 'You can't apply market forces to the care of the dying.'

End note: what happened to day care

Day care did not close down following its failure to gain a commitment from the Health Commission to fund it on a long-term basis. The NHS Trust and the Friends were placed in an extremely embarrassing situation: having successfully raised one million pounds from the local community, they were left with a building but no resources to finance its running costs. At the time, the Palliative Care Manager expressed her anxieties that 'we'll end up with a white elephant if we're not careful'. The NHS Trust provided a temporary reprieve by financing day care through its own limited charitable funds. A substantial, and unexpected, grant was then received from the Cancer Relief Macmillan Fund, which provided day care with full funding for the financial year 1996/1997 and partial funding for the following year. This grant was intended to create 'a breathing space in which a source of long-term funding must be sought' (cited from the Friend's Newsletter).

Following the Health Commission's response to the evaluation, staff became much stricter in discharging patients once their care packages came to an end. A decision was also made by NHS managers to change the name of the service from 'day care' to 'day therapy', in the hope that this would make it appear a more marketable commodity to NHS purchasers.

At the time of writing, all attempts to secure statutory funding for 'day therapy' had been abandoned. To prevent the closure of the service, the Friends appointed a professional fund-raiser in March 1998. Day care now survives on a day-to-day basis, relying entirely upon charitable donations from individuals and groups.

PREFACE TO CHAPTERS 3 AND 4

Changing contexts: entering the hospice

> Let's not pretend. This is not a happy place.
> (Joan – former day care patient, admitted to the hospice
> for symptom control)

> I now realise that I've been inadvertently spending a lot
> more time in day care than the hospice. ... The atmos-
> phere's so different between the two places. It's hard to put
> into words ... day care seems cheerful and full of life whilst
> the hospice seems stagnant and depressing.
> (Emma, volunteer co-ordinator for day care and the hospice)

The transition from day care to the hospice marked a radical change in my fieldwork. The hospice was only situated about a minute's walk away from day care but, as the comments above suggest, it was a very different kind of place: day care was a location for 'living', the hospice a space for 'dying'.

It is hard not to think of the time I spent in day care as a kind of 'utopian' encounter, since its strategies for masking deterioration were so effective. Yet the reality was that patients did deteriorate and, ultimately, they died. This, however, was really only brought home to me after I moved into the hospice, where the all-pervasive presence of deterioration, decline and death was impossible to avoid or deny.

Some of the patients I encountered in the hospice were people whom I had got to know well during my fieldwork in day care. I always felt some anxiety and trepidation when I recognised the name of a former day care patient who was just about to be admitted to the hospice. More often than not, such a feeling proved to be well-founded. On a number of occasions, I had to do a double take before being entirely confident that the patient I now saw curled up in bed was actually the person I had known from day care. Physical changes could be very noticeable and shocking: some patients experienced severe weight loss due to the ravaging effects of their cancer; others gained weight and became bloated as a result of being on steroids. Jaundice, with its characteristic yellowing of the skin and distinctive musty smell, was also fairly common.

Yet, in some respects, the physical changes I witnessed were considerably less distressing than the changes that seemed to have occurred in patients' moods and morale. A number of patients saw their admission to the hospice as occurring at a time when they had finally 'given up' and 'lost the will' to 'battle against' their illness. As Carla tearfully declared: 'I just don't have the energy to fight this thing anymore.' Another woman, Nancy, commented: 'Over the past couple of months I've gradually got weaker and weaker. ... Finally a course of chemotherapy totally knocked me out. I can't find the strength to do anything. ... I'm beyond caring. I doubt I'll leave this place alive.'

As I examine in the following chapters, many hospice patients had reached a stage in their illness at which they felt themselves to be 'taken over' by their diseased bodies: their bodily deterioration had an absolutely fundamental, non-negotiable impact upon their sense of self. The imagery of warfare, coupled with the patient's feeling that he or she had 'lost the battle' with his or her illness, are not coincidental.

It is hard to give a snapshot of what it was actually like to be in the hospice, because the atmosphere and the events taking place there changed substantially from one day to the next, and sometimes even within a matter of hours. Nevertheless, there are some general impressions that can be conveyed. I was, for example, always struck by the smell when I first walked into the building. It was not the typical antiseptic smell one would expect of a hospital setting; it was more pungent and nauseating: a combination of essential oils such as lemon and cinnamon, interlaced with the odour of vomit and excreta. Sometimes the smell was very strong, on other occasions it was much weaker; nonetheless, it was always there.

Coupled with the smell, there was an ubiquitous presence of bodily decay in the wards and side rooms – a presence which particularly shocked me on my first day of fieldwork, as the following extract from my fieldnotes suggests:

I found my first real encounter with the patients in the wards slightly repugnant. One of the beds we [another volunteer and myself] stripped down was covered in excreta. The woman concerned has MS and suffers from incontinence. ... A nurse was called into one of the cubicles to help out a woman who was vomiting. ... A man walked up and down the corridor with his penis and catheter hanging out through his pyjamas. Another woman lay on the top of her bed revealing a bloated stomach and scab covered legs.

The hospice was generally busiest in the mornings. This was the time when nurses rushed around the wards and side rooms, serving patients their breakfasts; administering their medications; giving patients bed baths and helping others to the bathroom or to get dressed. It was unusual for more than a handful of patients in the hospice to be ambulant and self-caring at any one time; most patients required substantial physical assistance with such things as getting into and out of bed and climbing onto and off a commode. Because so many patients required 'hands-on' care, nurses often complained that they were totally exhausted by the end of an early shift. Afternoons were normally more tranquil: some patients talked quietly to their visitors; others slept; still others sat in the chairs beside their beds, staring blankly into space, a distant and vacant look on their faces. Night times were generally even quieter, the silence punctuated only periodically by a patient talking or moaning in their sleep.

More often than not, one or more patients in the hospice lay in a ward or side room in a state of unconsciousness, their skeletal faces protruding above their bed clothes; their eyes glazed over; mouths gaping open; their breathing deep and erratic. Periodically a nurse would come to mop their brows and place a moistened sponge to their lips. It was only a question of time before such patients died, but the exact time of death was sometimes hard to predict; some remained in this state for a matter of hours, others for days. Meanwhile, relatives paced nervously up and down the corridors not knowing, it seemed, quite what to do with themselves: 'she's hanging on, only just ... when is it going to end?' Others chose to leave the hospice once a patient had slipped into a coma, their feeling being that their family member had already 'gone' (see Chapter 4).

Deaths that occurred in side rooms generally caused little in the way of a ripple within the hospice as a whole, because of the private nature of these locations. Deaths that took place in the wards, however, were extremely public events. In line with the modern hospice movement's ideology of an open confrontation with death, the curtains were normally kept open around a patient's bed throughout the period that they were in a coma. Activities on the ward continued as usual: nurses and volunteers milled around performing their routine tasks; visitors came and went; some patients slept, whilst others sat quietly in bed, the dying patient fully in their view. Nothing, it seemed, was kept hidden and secret. It was only after the patient had actually died that nursing staff finally drew the curtains around the bed. The other patients in the ward were informed of the death and invited to reflect upon their own feelings. Later the body was removed from the ward and taken to the viewing room to be laid out. Patients were normally asked if they wanted the curtains to be drawn around their own beds before the body was wheeled out. Most said 'yes'.

Within a setting in which there was such an overwhelming presence of deterioration and death, it is perhaps not too surprising that death, as a subject, was widely dwelt upon by patients. A death commonly prompted other patients in the ward to reflect upon their own deterioration and demise, often in an extremely open and direct manner:

> There were four of us in here and now there's only two ... and look at me, I'm not getting any better, am I? It will probably be my turn next.
>
> (Peggy)

> That man only came in last night and he's dead already [at the time, Robert was pointing to the empty space where the dead patient's bed had been]. At least he's at peace. I know what I've got ... provided they keep me free of pain I'll be happy.
>
> (Robert)

> Look at him. Poor old boy, it doesn't look like he's got long to go. Well, I guess that's what we're all in here for.
>
> (Brian)

When patients talked about their own imminent deaths their words did not, as a general rule, indicate any obvious sense of anger. Yet the opposite – a peaceful state of acceptance (see

Kübler-Ross 1969) – also seemed to be absent. The overwhelming impression I gained from patients was that their feelings were those of dulled resignation; of apathy, lethargy and exhaustion; of finally giving up.

Behind the scenes, a different and more emotionally volatile picture emerged. As I indicated in Chapter 1, my fieldwork took place during a somewhat turbulent period, since the recent changes that had occurred in the Health Commission's funding of the region's palliative care services had had a substantial impact upon the hospice and the working practices taking place within it. Bed cutbacks, in particular, undermined staff's morale significantly, exacerbating the rift that existed between them and the NHS management. Staff's low morale and, inevitably, anger became particularly evident in the context of the once-weekly multi-disciplinary meetings where patient 'caseloads' were discussed. After a further three beds had been cut in the hospice, the issue of patient discharges came to predominate these meetings, much to the resentment and disillusionment of some staff members. Exchanges in multi-disciplinary meetings often became very bitter, with staff complaining that they were under such pressure to empty beds that they were sometimes forced to discharge patients against their own wishes. As the physiotherapist shouted out on one occasion, 'gone are the days when we could call this place a hospice'. Shortly before I actually started my fieldwork, low morale, anger and disillusionment amongst staff had become so extreme that several members of the nursing team resigned. A couple of other members of staff were also on long-term sick leave. It is important to recognise that it was against this somewhat turbulent back-drop that the fieldwork I now go on to describe was conducted.

3

'BODY-SUBJECT' TO 'BODY-OBJECT'

Hospice care and the dying patient

> Cancer is often referred to as the 'illness of modern civiliza-
> tion,' referring to the toxicity of our environment, physical
> and mental. But cancer may also be an illness of our cen-
> tury in defying science's efforts to control decay, suffering,
> the body, and death. For the body in cancer is not the fa-
> mous docile one – to the contrary. It is the body asserting
> itself, out of control of its 'owners' and 'curers,' on its own,
> producing its own monsters that science and medicine are
> called upon to control.
>
> (Gordon 1990: 292)

Introduction

This chapter develops the theme of the body in illness and,
ultimately, in death which, as Gordon observes, may elude the
control both of its owner and those participating in a patient's care.
The following discussions will highlight the non-negotiability of a
patient's deteriorating body in his or her experiences of self and in
the dialectical processes through which his or her identity is
constructed and evaluated within the wider social context. As we
shall see, as patients lost the ability to act as the agents of their
embodied actions, a fundamental loss of self occurred; a situation
which confounds Cartesian notions of a mind–body duality. For
patients close to death (particularly for those with cancer) this
process of change and loss was experienced in an especially sharp
and painful manner; physical and mental deterioration often being
very rapid at this stage. The early part of this chapter will serve as a
critique of the existing literature on the body and embodiment
which, as I hope to show, has not entirely succeeded in bringing the
body as a material, physically experienced phenomenon into social

analysis. The chapter then goes on to highlight and explore the intersubjective impact a patient's bodily deterioration may have upon family and friends involved with his or her 'hands-on' care. The chapter concludes by pointing to some difficulties inherent within the ideological tenet central to the hospice movement of enabling patients to 'live until they die'. Whilst the movement aims to sustain a patient's selfhood to the point of physical death, the material outlined here will suggest that hospice care is, in reality, both constrained by, and reinforces, an identity in a deteriorating patient wherein she or he is progressively reduced from what I term a 'body-subject' to a 'body-object'.

The body and embodiment: existing paradigms

There is now an increasing number of ethnographic and theoretical studies which challenge sociology's and anthropology's hitherto 'disembodied' view of its subject. Thanks largely to the far-ranging influence of the work of Foucault, anthropologists and sociologists have started to recognise the general absence of the body from most writing (see, for example, Turner 1984, 1992; Shilling 1993). Indeed, as Lock has observed, it is only comparatively recently that researchers have stopped 'bracketing' the body 'as a black box' which is then 'set aside' (1993: 133). There are, nonetheless, some obvious exceptions to this earlier trend, most notably perhaps, Douglas' extensive treatment and analysis of the body as a 'symbol of society' and as a 'cultural text' (1970, 1984).[1] Within Douglas' social classificatory approach, however, the materiality of the body is side-stepped, a situation which is also evident in other symbolic and metaphoric analyses such as those of Hertz (1960) and Victor Turner (1967). As Csordas suggests, approaches such as these typically 'study the *body* and its transformations while still taking *embodiment* for granted' (1994: 6, original emphasis). Jackson, likewise, argues that these particular studies tend 'to be overtly symbolic and semantic' (1989: 122), reducing the body to the status of a sign (1989: 123). Hence, the more recent approaches to the body and embodiment have been concerned with 're-embodying' the subject by incorporating the body as a lived, 'flesh and bones' entity into their academic frameworks of analysis.

In criticising traditional sociological approaches for treating the body as an 'absent presence', a presence which is generally taken as implicit rather than made explicit in sociological accounts (Shilling 1993), academics have challenged the idea that the body is a fixed material entity, 'existing prior to the mutability and flux of cultural change and diversity' (Csordas 1994: 1). It has, to the contrary, now been widely argued that there is no 'natural' body that exists outside culture (Frank 1993; Falk 1995), and hence the body and experiences of embodiment must be examined and understood within their full cultural context (Mascia-Lees and Sharpe 1992). Indeed, writers who have examined contemporary 'Western' modes of embodiment have pointed to a number of culturally and historically-specific, interdependent variables which, they suggest, have given rise to the idea of the body as a central locus and vehicle for the self within this particular milieu. The variables highlighted include the forces of secularisation; the rise of ascetic individualism (Crawford 1994; Giddens 1991; Shilling 1993); and the development of narcissistic and hedonistic consumer culture (Featherstone 1993; Featherstone *et al.* 1993; Falk 1994).[2]

A common theme emerging from these accounts is the idea that the body of modern 'Western' contexts has become a medium through which the self is shaped, fashioned and expressed (Giddens 1991). This conception is aptly summarised by Shilling who suggests that the contemporary 'Western' body has become 'a *project* which should be worked at and accomplished as part of an *individual's* self-identity' (1993: 5, original emphasis; see also Coward 1989). Underlying this notion is the idea of the 'performing self' of appearance, display and impression management (Goffman 1959; Featherstone 1993: 187), expressed and achieved through a body which acts as a source of 'physical/cultural capital' (Bourdieu 1984).[3] Thus, as Crossley argues, the body and embodied action provide 'the information upon which judgements about self-hood and moral worth are made' (1995: 139). Likewise, Bordo, in her study of eating disorders and body building, suggests that the body has increasingly become 'a site of individual self-determination' (1993: 20) serving the purpose of social mobility within a culture in which the appearance of the outer body has 'come to operate as a market of personal, internal order ... as a symbol for the emotional, moral or spiritual state of the individual' (1993: 193). Crawford similarly suggests that the healthy body has 'become a sign of individual achievement ... [it] is the mark of distinction that differentiates those who deserve to succeed from those who will fail' (1994: 1354).

What is clearly suggested in approaches such as these is that the modern 'Western' body does not simply constitute a site for the inscription of the values of late modernity: as Benson argues in her discussion of practices such as body-building and tattooing, ideas of the body as 'property'; as a thing 'owned' and 'fashioned' by the self, have also become central to contemporary experiences of embodiment (Benson 1996).[4]

The above accounts thus attempt to bring the body of the modern 'West' into the picture by highlighting ways in which selfhood is fashioned and expressed both through, and within, the medium of corporeality. Yet is the body really made fully visible within these scholarly works? It is one of my contentions in this chapter that the majority of recent approaches to the body are extremely problematic because most appear to take for granted the presence of a healthy, autonomously functioning body; that is, of a body which can actually be 'controlled' and 'fashioned' by the self. The other side of the coin, namely, the diseased body and flesh; the body that places physical and material constraints upon the self, has received considerably less attention. Indeed, even where the body in illness is allegedly given centre stage, as in much of the literature within medical anthropology and medical sociology, it is not (usually) the body as a material and experiential entity which is the focus but, rather, the emphasis has tended to remain on the social and cultural consequences of affliction.[5] As a result, although some studies do recognise that the body can become a 'problem' in chronic illness and old age (Featherstone and Hepworth 1993: 173; Williams 1996) and in death (Shilling 1993: 175) precisely because of the 'emphasis that many modern individuals place on their bodies as constitutive of the self' (1993: 182), the exact impact of bodily deterioration upon selfhood remains, as the sociologists Kelly and Field (1996) have observed, to be satisfactorily explored. Clearly, this particular ethnographic study is now very timely.

This chapter will cast the relationship between body and self in a new light by making the deteriorating, 'non-negotiable' bodies of dying patients the central focus of both observation and analysis. Consideration will be paid to the subjective experiences of patients themselves, and to the various ways in which such experiences are mediated and affected by the wider social and cultural context. In so doing, I will show that having the *bodily* ability to negotiate and alter one's environment is a crucial aspect of person/self in contemporary English contexts; an aspect, furthermore, which really only becomes visible after it has been lost (see also Leder 1990; Williams 1996).

Indeed, there are strong grounds for suggesting that this aspect of embodiment has remained implicit, perhaps even invisible, in most of the accounts of the body because they have been written for, and by, young(ish) intellectuals who can take their mobility and autonomy for granted. As Leder notes, for persons for whom the body functions unproblematically, the body tends to disappear from conscious awareness (1990: 3), it becomes, as it were, a form of 'experiential absence' (1990: 2), a phenomenon which, as he further observes, 'plays a crucial role in encouraging and supporting Cartesian dualism' (1990: 3). A similar observation has been made by Diprose who notes that (for the healthy and 'ablebodied'), 'in our ordinary, everyday activities, our body is open upon a world and engaged with it in such a way that we are hardly aware of this body at all' (1995: 209; see also Csordas 1994: 8). Thus, as she further suggests, 'I do not direct my body to act. For the most part my body and the world with which it is engaged, are not objects for my attention' (ibid.).

It is perhaps not too surprising, therefore, that it has been left to a small minority of academics, most typically those reflecting upon their own experiences of bodily dysfunction and deterioration, to throw such taken-for-granted aspects of embodiment into question. As the social anthropologist Robert Murphy suggests:

> People in good health take their lot, and their bodies, for granted; they can see, hear, eat, make love and breathe because they have working organs that can do all of those things. ... Each person simply accepts the fact that he [*sic*] has two legs and can walk; he does not think about it or marvel at it any more than he would feel gratitude for the oxygen content of air. These are among the simple existential conditions of life ... illness [however] negates this lack of awareness of the body in guiding our thought and actions. The body can no longer be taken for granted, implicit and axiomatic, for it has become a problem.
>
> (Murphy 1987: 11–12)

Murphy was writing of his own experience of a gradually expanding tumour in his spine which led first to paraplegia, and eventually, over a number of years, to quadriplegia and the reduction of his mobility 'to a vegetal state' (1987: 149) (as Murphy also recognised, the tumour would ultimately cause him to die). What his account begins to draw our attention towards here are both the 'visibility' and the 'non-negotiability' of the deteriorating physical body; of the body which ceases to be 'plastic' and controlled by the self.[6] Yet whilst Murphy's work is important in highlighting the contingent nature of the self in the face of bodily deterioration (and, indeed, the contingency of the body itself (see Leder 1990)), there are grounds for arguing that his study is only of limited applicability. A notable feature of Murphy's account is that, in the process of losing the bodily ability to command and move through space, he experienced to some extent a 'redefinition' of self which involved a shift in emphasis away from bodily to mental capacities (Thomas Couser 1997: 185). As Murphy described in the final pages of his book, 'my thoughts and sense of being alive have been [progressively] driven back into my brain, where I now reside' (1987: 187). Thus, whilst Murphy is very clear that his 'status as a member of society' diminished after his body degenerated (1987: 3), he was, nonetheless, able to retain a viable sense of self even after his bodily deterioration had become very severe. (Indeed, this phenomenon is made only too apparent by the fact that he both wanted to, and did, successfully write a highly reflexive study of the social, personal and theoretical issues that surrounded his illness.) What one has to question here is the extent to which the experiences and self-conceptions Murphy shares with his audience can be thought of as typical of people suffering from severe loss of bodily mobility as a whole. Thomas Couser, in his study of illness, disability and life writing, makes the valuable point that autobiographical and auto-ethnographical accounts of illness and disability (such as Murphy's) are likely to be 'best-case scenarios' because 'those who undertake autobiography tend to be intellectuals, whose major sources of self-esteem – and income – are less likely to be damaged by physical disability' (1997: 205).[7] Thus, as he further points out, 'the redemptive shifting of emphasis from the body to the mind' (1997: 185) typically experienced and described by these writers may be somewhat unusual; it could quite possibly stem from the fact that 'their intellectual power was able to compensate for their loss of physical power and control of their lower bodies' (ibid.). In most cases, he suggests, 'illness or disability may turn people so far inward that they become virtual black holes, absorbing energy rather than emitting illumination' (1997: 5). Consequently, 'the conditions that may stimulate autobiographical reflection' (by heightening consciousness of self and contingency, for example), may 'also obstruct its expression'; chronic disability can annihilate selfhood (ibid.).

The observations developed in the following pages would certainly seem to support such an argument. The account that follows describes the experiences of patients who received care in the hospice during their last weeks and days of life. In the final stages approaching death, these patients often underwent a very rapid deterioration in their strength, dexterity and therefore bodily mobility: a phenomenon which cast the relationship between body and self in a new, often in very graphic ways. Unlike patients at an earlier stage in their illness (such as those who attended day care), and patients with long-term disabilities and chronic conditions (see, for example, Seymour 1998; Charmaz 1991, 1995a), hospice patients did not have time, or a context, in which to mask and/or reconfigure their bodily deterioration, and thereby 'remake' a self (see my discussion of the use of prosthetic devices later on in this chapter). The deteriorating body, and its effects upon the self, thus became visible in a very stark form.

In exploring the impact of bodily deterioration upon the self, the analysis which follows will make extensive use of the phenomenological notion of the 'lived body', as developed by Sartre (1956) and Merleau-Ponty (1962). From a phenomenological perspective, a person is not embodied in the sense that they 'have' a body, but in the sense that they 'exist' or 'live' their body (Toombs 1995). The body as it is 'lived' thus represents a person's particular point of view on the world; it is the body that is the vehicle for seeing (Merleau-Ponty 1962: 90). As such, 'the subject that I am, when taken concretely, is inseparable from this body and this world' (1962: 408). Understanding embodiment as the experience of both being a body, and living through a body, thus provides an important conceptual perspective for understanding why a patient's self is affected when various bodily capacities and capabilities are lost. In this chapter, as I have already indicated, the central focus will be upon patients' 'lived experience' (Jackson 1996: 2) of loss of bodily mobility. A similar theme will also be developed in the following chapter which examines a special case of loss of bodily autonomy: the loss of control of the physical boundaries of the body.

The 'dying' patient: transition from 'subject' to 'object'

A significant feature of advanced cancer in its late stages is the rapid deterioration it can induce in a patient's bodily strength and physical dexterity. The development of bone secondaries can be especially debilitating because they cause the bones to become very brittle and hence to break easily. Similarly, the development and spread of cancer within the lungs may severely restrict mobility since patients find that even the slightest physical exertion results in their becoming extremely breathless. Tim, for example, had to pass his days and nights sitting rigidly upright in the chair beside his bed. He explained that if he moved suddenly, or lay down horizontally, he felt as if he were drowning: 'It's like diving too deep into a swimming pool and then finding you can't get back to the surface in time. It's so scary.'

Accelerating weakness and lethargy also resulted from other bodily dysfunctions such as anaemia or the failure of organs like the liver, kidneys and pancreas. A small proportion of patients developed a spinal cord compression[8] leading to paraplegia, sometimes very suddenly. For instance, Millie was walking down the stairs in her home when, all at once, her legs gave way beneath her. She was admitted to the hospice the following day and remained bed-bound until she died. Other patients developed gross oedema in their legs and arms. Lymph fluid would accumulate in their limbs causing them to become very heavy and swollen. Consequently, these patients became severely restricted in their bodily ability to move through space.

It was not uncommon for patients to be admitted to the hospice whilst still able to walk (granted, sometimes only a few paces without assistance) only to discover that within a matter of days their weakness was such that even the simplest of acts such as lifting a cup to their lips had become too strenuous. Thus, as patients deteriorated, they ceased to be the agents of their own actions, becoming progressively more and more dependent upon others for their immediate bodily care. Many required help with washing and using the commode, some needed to be hoisted in order to be moved from chair to bed, while others required assistance with feeding. As one newly bed-bound patient put it simply, 'now all of you will have to do everything for me'.

The impact that this type of bodily deterioration had upon a patient's self was incisively highlighted by Frank, when he reflected upon his own experiences. Frank originally developed cancer in his prostate, but it spread to his bones and then to his lungs. A few weeks prior to his admission for respite care his mobility had decreased substantially. Up to that point, Frank had been independent, ambulant and able to attend to his own bodily care, but by the time he came into the hospice he could only manage to walk very short distances independently and required help with washing and using the toilet. He spent most of his time sitting in the chair beside his bed with an oxygen cylinder close at hand for when he became very breathless. As he suggested:

> For me the physical and mental are entwined. I've found as I've got weaker I've become a lot more apathetic and withdrawn. ... I've abandoned a lot of my favourite pastimes. A couple of months ago I stopped doing the crossword in the newspaper. Last month I stopped reading the newspaper altogether. I've just lost interest. I suppose that's why so many patients here spend so much time sleeping. There's so few things we're able to do ... so you just *give up*.
>
> (Frank, emphasis added)

As Frank's comments suggest, patients did not generally experience their deteriorating bodies in terms of alienation or dissociation; there was no simple separation or preservation of the 'I' or 'me' in a 'mind' disassociated from the body. On the contrary, as Frank indicated in his own words, the 'physical' and the 'mental' are fundamentally linked. I noticed that as their bodily strength and mobility deteriorated significantly, many hospice patients experienced what appeared to be a tangential loss of self. Such a phenomenon differed from the 'total loss of self' (evinced as a mental switching off) observed amongst some of the 'unbounded' patients described in the next chapter. Rather, the patients considered here experienced what Toombs (1995) has described as 'existential fatigue' and an 'impetus to withdraw' in her exploration of the 'lived experience' of degenerative conditions such as multiple sclerosis. As she suggests:

> The effortful nature of worldly involvement that is characteristic of incapacitating disorders can engender a sense of fatigue that I shall call 'existential fatigue.' To organise and carry out projects requires not only physical ability but, as importantly, an exercise of will. When ceaseless and ongoing effort is required to perform the simplest of tasks (getting out of bed, dressing, taking a shower, going on a trip), there is a powerful impulse to withdraw, to cease doing what is required. Consequently, physical incapacity exerts a centripetal force in another sense. The person with

a disability is tempted severely to curtail involvements in the world.

(Toombs 1995: 15)

Many of those patients who remained sentient and lucid until their deaths occurred did continue to communicate, but the nature of their conversations suggested that they had, like Frank, experienced an erosion of self. Such a phenomenon was made particularly evident by Geoff, a bed-bound patient, who wryly suggested that it must be extremely difficult to engage patients in conversations for research because: 'After all, most of us in here have gone past the stage where we're into in-depth conversations about the meaning of life and all that willy-nilly.'

Geoff's insights often proved to be accurate. In strong contrast to the situation in day care, I did encounter substantial difficulties in coaxing many weak and immobile patients into discussing matters which extended beyond mundane topics such as the weather (a difficulty, I should add, which was also shared by visitors, staff and volunteers). It could be argued, nonetheless, that this is a significant finding in itself: the problems I (and others) experienced would seem to indicate that many patients had already become, to some degree, stripped of who they were.

Since it frequently proved difficult to encourage patients to participate in conversations and research interviews, direct observation of their behaviour provided an alternative, and often more viable, means of studying their 'lived experience' of bodily deterioration. Indeed, Crossley, in his synthesis of the work of Merleau-Ponty and Goffman, argues convincingly that behaviour is 'simultaneously meaningful, embodied and intelligent' (1995: 143), since 'the mindedness and embodiment of human life are inseparable' (ibid.). Hence, as he further suggests, 'the subjective or mental states of others are available to us, directly, and ours ... are available to them, directly, in the form of our behaviours; subjectivity is not private and inaccessible, it is worldly and publicly available' (1995: 143).

Patient behaviour, which was characterised by staff as 'apathy' and 'withdrawal', was an issue of ongoing concern within the hospice. Such a phenomenon was clearly central to the day room 'problem' that staff hoped I would address when I began my fieldwork. Shortly before I started my research, the five bed ward which had been closed down was converted into a day room (see Chapter 1). This new day room was intended to mirror the functions of day care, with a part-time occupational therapist, assisted by volunteers, offering a menu of relaxation sessions, craft and other therapeutic activities to patients. The intention was to provide them with a source of social stimulation which was in line with the formal hospice philosophy of enabling patients 'to live until they die'. In spite of persistent efforts by staff to coax patients into spending time in the day room, I observed that attendance remained consistently low throughout the duration of my fieldwork. 'I can't be bothered' or 'I'd rather rest' were the most typical responses patients offered for wishing to remain within the immediate vicinity of their beds. In fact, the factor most likely to encourage patients to spend time in the day room was when a particularly distressing death was occurring in their ward.

Disengagement and loss of self became evident not only in patients' lack of interest in, and withdrawal from, opportunities for social interaction, but also in their changing relationship to their personal possessions. This phenomenon is well illustrated in the case of Penny, who was admitted to the hospice with chronic obstructive airways disease (COAD). Penny was one of the more atypical patients I encountered during research: firstly, because the nature of her illness meant that her trajectory of deterioration was significantly slower than most of the other patients; and, secondly, because of her home circumstances – she was resident in the hospice for almost five months (until she died), apart from two brief visits home.[9] I was thus able to work very closely with Penny over a comparatively extended period of time.

When Penny was first admitted she was bed-bound, but retained strength and dexterity in her arms and hands. Hence, she was still able to pursue several of her favourite pastimes such as knitting, reading books and doing jigsaws. At this point, she was active, engaged and extremely talkative. As she settled into the hospice she surrounded herself with an increasing number of personal possessions, brought in for her by her family. Penny's corner of the ward – 'Santa's grotto' as the staff jokingly called it – was piled with framed photographs of her grandchildren, cuddly toys, potted plants and several ornaments from home.

After a couple of months, Penny's condition began to deteriorate. She had an attack of angina and then developed a chest infection. As a consequence, her weakness and lethargy increased substantially and she lost most of the strength in her arms. As she became more unwell, Penny expressed the wish to spend some time at home before she died, and staff were able to organise twenty-four-hour nursing cover for a week. The morning she was readmitted, she had a further severe attack of angina, which left her so weak that she was unable to do anything for herself, though she could still talk with effort. Staff expressed their sadness that she had lost the last vestiges of her independence: Penny had to abandon all of her favourite pastimes and was even unable to administer her own medication.

Her family had returned all of her personal possessions with her to the hospice, but when nursing staff started to arrange them around her bedside she told them not to bother, suggesting that they put them into a large bag in the cupboard outside the ward instead. The following day, she asked me to remove her handbag from her locker and empty the contents onto the bed. These included a large number of family photos and personal letters (some with 1940s postmarks). Penny told me to tear up all of the letters and throw them away. She also asked me to take the photos and place them in the same bag as her other possessions. She did not look at them again. The shedding of these personal possessions (many of which had a long history and could thus be associated with her memory and past) was Penny's last obvious act of authorship. She did not actually die until about a month later. At the time of her death, she was surrounded by nothing but a couple of get well cards.

A wide corpus of literature posits a close connection between consumption behaviour, selfhood and identity in contemporary 'Western' contexts. The work of various writers suggests that consumption is eminently social, relational and active, rather than private, atomic and passive. Consumption, it is argued, involves the translation of the alienable into the inalienable, of use-values into sign-values. Thus personal possessions become attachable to their owners (Miller 1988, 1991; Appadurai 1986), and serve as signs by which people relate to one another (Douglas and Isherwood 1979) and negotiate and display their social status (Baudrillard 1981). Hence there are strong grounds for arguing that personal items and other consumption goods are closely interlinked with the construction and expression of selfhood. Letters, photographs and other items of sentimental value are, for many people, especially closely bound up with this process.

Such an analytical perspective suggests that patients' declining attachment to personal possessions, as their bodies weakened, may be taken as a further indication of a loss of self that many had experienced. Particularly pertinent in Penny's case is the fact that she dissociated herself from all items of personal and sentimental value at more or less the same time as she completely lost the bodily ability to act as the agent of her actions and intentions. Penny's behaviour was not atypical in this regard: it was extremely unusual for 'high-dependency' patients – especially those admitted for terminal care – to bring personal items with them into the hospice, in spite of staff's encouragement for them to do so (staff believed that such items would help to reinforce a home and family atmosphere). In contrast, respite patients, especially those who retained their mobility, characteristically surrounded themselves with items of sentimental value, particularly photographs of family.[10] Helen, for example, was admitted for a week's respite, and, on her admission, covered the walls around her bed with photos of herself, her partner and their children. She also asked her partner to bring in a series of paintings by her youngest daughter. By surrounding herself with images of 'life', she made a clear statement about her continued perception of herself as a wife and mother; as a person with active and significant relations to others.

One might be tempted to argue that patients behaved in the ways just described because they had entered, and were enacting, a 'dying role' (see, for example, Field 1996; Seale 1998). If that were the case, it could be further suggested that patients were in fact exhibiting a changed self, rather than a loss of self as such. Yet such a position is problematic on two accounts in particular. First, and perhaps most obviously, because the behaviour of the vast majority of patients did not actually conform to the 'scripts' associated with the 'dying role', the latter being portrayed in both revivalist discourse and the media as an heroic event, an intense 'creative activity' and a 'fight' until the end (see Seale 1998).[11] Indeed, it is not only the modern hospice movement that has propagated this conception of 'living until one dies' (see Chapter 1), the stereotype also has much broader resonance; for example, in Hollywood deathbed scenes. And the fact that patients' behaviour did not concur with these wider social stereotypes brings us to the second and more fundamental point: their apathy and withdrawal appeared to stem primarily from their declining ability to act in embodied ways, rather than from a knowledge of impending death *per se*. Such a phenomenon has already been highlighted in the observations and analyses above, yet it came out most clearly in the metaphors patients used to describe themselves and to construct and rationalise their current experiences.

As the work of Lakoff and Johnson suggests, the metaphors that emerge in day-to-day interactions provide a particularly valuable avenue for accessing experiences and conceptions of self, since metaphors are employed in everyday language both to construct and reflect subjective reality. As they describe:

> In all aspects of life … we define our reality in terms of metaphors and then proceed to act on the basis of the metaphors. We draw inferences, set goals, make commitments, and execute plans, all on the basis of how we in part structure our experience, consciously and unconsciously, by means of metaphor.
>
> (Lakoff and Johnson 1980: 158)

Jackson, in a similar vein, has suggested that 'metaphors evoke and mediate connections within experience' (1996: 9; see also Fernandez 1977). What is particularly striking about my observations is that, as patients' physical weakness and degree of dependency increased, the metaphors they employed to describe themselves commonly shifted from those relating to a 'subject' to those relating to an 'object'. This was especially apparent in the very high frequency of references patients made to becoming a 'burden' and to other inert, redundant, object-like states. Such metaphors thus not only indicated a loss of self on the part of 'high-dependency' patients, but, more importantly still, an 'interdependency of body and mind, self and world' (Jackson 1996: 9): the 'object' evoked was not the body as such but, rather, the patient him or herself. Thus, whilst there may be a certain validity to Leder's suggestion that: 'Insofar as the body seizes our awareness at times of disturbance, it can appear "Other" and opposed to the self' (1990: 70), the seeming appearance of a Cartesian dualism is somewhat deceptive. What one has to take into account is that the very aspects of the body that become visible during periods of dysfunction may, at the same time, have a fundamental, debasing impact upon the self.

Indeed it is noteworthy that all the patients in this study made a direct connection between their 'object-like' self conceptions and the loss of mobility which had ensued through their deterioration. Ann, for example, who was admitted to the hospice for symptom control, became wheelchair-bound during her stay. The strength and dexterity of her arms also decreased substantially. As a consequence, she required the assistance of two nurses to lift her in and out of bed and onto and off the commode. As she put it:

There's absolutely no point in me going home unless I can get from a chair to my bed. I can't do anything any more. I'd just be *one big burden* on my family.

(Ann, emphasis added)

Similarly, a bed-bound male patient, George, admitted for terminal care, commented:

I can't do anything for myself any more. I can't help others. I'm a *useless burden*; I'm just a *waste of space*.

(George, emphasis added)

Another woman, Joy, had advanced MS and came into the hospice for respite care after her husband had a minor heart attack and required hospital treatment. Joy had no mobility in her arms and legs and required help with feeding. She frequently referred to herself as 'useless' and apologised for being 'too much trouble'. On one occasion, I took her to hospital in a wheelchair to visit her husband. On our way out, she commented that he looked much better because, 'I'm not bothering him anymore'. She then suggested that I threw her out of the nearest window. We were on the sixth floor at the time.

As their comments indicate, one of the most common reasons patients expressed for either wanting to be admitted to the hospice, or for remaining there, was because of their anxieties of being 'too much of a burden' on those family members and friends who would have to care for them back at home. Patients often openly suggested that, by coming into the hospice, they considered the welfare of their family as being more important than their own (note the lack of self-interest here). This situation was brought home to me very movingly by Roz, whom I had talked to frequently whilst I was conducting fieldwork in day care. During one frank interview at that time, Roz spoke very openly of her fear of the hospice: 'You'll never get me into a place like that'. She made it very clear that she wanted to die at home rather than spending her last days 'in that death factory watching the other patients drop off like flies'. I met Roz again about a year later, just after she had been admitted to the hospice for terminal care. As soon as she recognised me, an emotional outpouring began:

It was okay until a couple of days ago, when I could still walk with a frame. Then suddenly my legs gave way beneath me. The next thing I knew I was lying flat on the carpet in the living room. I couldn't move, and my husband couldn't help me up. I was lying there for such a long time. I'm sure the imprint from my body must still be there. In the end he had to get a neighbour to help lift me up.

Roz went on to tell me that, after this incident, she had waited until her husband had gone out of the house to do some shopping and then rang up the hospice and 'begged the staff' to admit her. I expressed some surprise after recalling the vehemence of the comments she had made a year previously. Roz put me in the picture:

> I've come in here more for my husband than myself. *What I want doesn't really matter that much anymore anyway. I've become such a burden.* He had to give up his job seven weeks ago to help care for me. He's reached the end of his tether. When I had the fall I knew he couldn't cope. So, yes, I've done it for him, I suppose. It's not fair *to drag him down with me* any longer.
>
> (Roz, emphasis added)

Roz's weakness accelerated within twenty-four hours of her admission. She died in the hospice a few days later.

The patient as 'object': shifts in temporal perspectives

> By considering the body in movement, we can see better how it inhabits space (and, moreover, time) because movement is not limited to submitting passively to space and time, it actively assumes them, it takes them up in their basic significance which is obscured in the commonplaceness of established situations.
>
> (Merleau-Ponty 1962: 102)

The experiences of high-dependency patients as 'static', 'body-objects' was further reflected and reinforced in their subjective constructions and perceptions of space and time. As the quote from Merleau-Ponty suggests, embodiment as a mode of being-in-the-world and, by implication, one's bodily ability to control and command space, impinges directly upon one's temporal perspectives: motion 'encompasses simultaneously position, temporality and identity' (Langer 1989: 85). A similar argument has been made by Ardener who suggests that time and space are mutually affecting spheres of reality, 'where "reality" is understood to depend upon human apperceptions' (1981: 15). Such analytical perspectives would suggest that a loss of bodily mobility would be accompanied by a changing perception of space and time; a phenomenon which did indeed appear to occur amongst the hospice patients with whom I worked. As I now go on to explore, as patients' bodies became reduced to a progressively 'inert state', their constructions and perceptions of space and time also appeared to become increasingly bounded and static.

Shrinking spaces

To return to the day room problem discussed earlier, there are some grounds for suggesting that patients' reluctance to use this particular room did not result solely from their declining interest in participating in recreational activities and interacting with others; it also stemmed from a more general anxiety about moving (or being moved) away from the immediate vicinity of their beds. What constituted a 'safe space' for patients appeared to be dictated by their own bodily capabilities: large and unfamiliar places (such as the day room) were experienced as intimidating and frightening by patients with poor mobility because these patients were severely constricted in their bodily ability to command and negotiate such space. Kirsty, for example, had advanced MS and was admitted to the hospice for a two-week period of respite to allow her partner and children to go away on holiday. She asked to be put into a side room because she had witnessed a particularly distressing death in the ward she had stayed in during her previous stay. About a week into her admission, staff became concerned that she was feeling isolated and alone in her single room, a problem which was heightened by the fact that her family were not around to visit her. Nursing staff encouraged her to spend some time in the day room, suggesting that she might 'enjoy a change of scenery'. Kirsty was dressed and put into a wheelchair and taken to the day room where the TV was switched on for her to watch. Because she had no mobility in her arms, she could not use a buzzer to notify staff if she needed assistance. One of the nurses, consequently, asked me to go into the day room regularly to check and see if Kirsty needed anything. I made my first visit about half an hour later and discovered her in a state of extreme anxiety. She said she felt 'terrified' and 'helpless' and asked me to take her back to her side room immediately. Kirsty, at the time, found it hard to explain why she had found being in the day room such a daunting experience. A little later on in the day, however, she suggested that, 'being there made me feel like a tiny fish in a gigantic ocean'. She refused to leave her single room for the remainder of her stay in the hospice.

For some patients, spaces and places within the hospice which had been familiar haunts on previous stays became, at a later stage in their deterioration, unfamiliar and daunting terrain. Michael, for example, made several visits to the hospice for pain control after he developed bone secondaries (he was originally diagnosed as having cancer of the bladder). During his early stays in the hospice, he was mobile and independent, though his repeated bouts of pain were a source of considerable demoralisation and distress to him: Michael often likened the sensation of pain he experienced to 'sitting on a sharp knife'. He was extremely anxious to do anything he could to keep his mind off the pain and, consequently, spent most of his time in the tea room at the front of the hospice because this created numerous opportunities to chat to visitors (normally those making visits to other patients) as well as to staff and volunteers who regularly passed by.

Michael's pain control was finally successfully sorted out, and he was able to return home for several months. He was readmitted after bone secondaries had spread to his jaw causing new problems with pain. By this stage, he had also deteriorated significantly: his cancer had spread to his lungs and liver and he had become wheelchair-bound.

On his readmission, Michael was extremely subdued and spent the first few days sitting quietly in the chair beside his bed. The nurses noticed that he had become very withdrawn and decided to try to 'perk him up' by taking him to the tea bar in his wheelchair; this particular place, as they pointed out, had been his favourite haunt during his previous stays in the hospice. I was asked to escort Michael along with another nurse. As soon as we left the confines of the ward, Michael became very anxious; he grabbed hold of my hand and clasped it firmly whilst the nurse pushed him along the corridor. When we entered the tea bar, his sense of panic heightened and he started to hyperventilate. The nurse and I tried to calm him down, but to no avail: 'Please take me back! It doesn't look the same. ... I'm not the same. I've never been this bad before.' We returned Michael to the safety of his own bed where, as he later pointed out, 'I feel in control ... everything I need's within easy reach' (he was pointing to his glasses and the drink beside his bed at the time). Such an incident illustrates a 'shrinkage' that had occurred in the spaces in which patients, such as Michael, felt safe. Yet this particular encounter was, for him at least, also a painful and graphic reminder of the things he was no longer able to do for himself; of the person he no longer was.

Static time

In exploring hospice patients' changed perceptions of time, a particularly notable contrast can be drawn with day care patients. As I discussed in Chapter 2, many day care patients maintained a sense of self by distancing themselves from their uncertain and unpredictable futures, pushing the concept of the future into the realm of the abstract. In addition, patients constructed a stable 'autobiography of self' in the present by using the past as a reservoir from which positive events could be drawn and relationships with others imagined and reinvoked. A similar phenomenon occurs amongst the elderly. Rowles, for example, points to a plethora of gerontological research indicating, 'a propensity for increasing "interiority", reminiscence, and a process of life review among the elderly' (1980: 60). This process, he suggests, expresses 'an accommodation to growing old which, for the participants, provided liberation from the time–space constrictions of personal decline' (ibid.).

Deteriorating hospice patients, in contrast, appeared to have disengaged themselves not only from their futures but also from their pasts. I was struck by the fact that it was extremely unusual for 'high-dependency' patients to make references to aspects of their lives prior to their admission to the hospice, even when they were encouraged to reminisce or talk about their former careers. Yet such a pattern of dissociation became perhaps most evident in an event which took place on VE Day in 1995, when national celebrations marked the fiftieth anniversary of the end of World War II in Europe. The newly appointed volunteer co-ordinator decided to mark the occasion by organising a tea party in the day room and wards: many of the hospice patients were over 60, so she thought that memories of the war would be important to them. The whole of the building was decorated, cakes purchased and a Max Bygraves video ordered for a 'sing along'. A distinct wave of apathy hit the hospice as soon as the party was scheduled to start. Only two patients participated, and both had brain tumours, and were considered by the nurses to be more or less unaware of their environment. The other patients remained staunchly in their side rooms and wards, even ignoring the television events being broadcast at the time. Fortunately, one of the nurses had the good sense to extend a last-minute invitation to a number of elderly women from the geriatric unit located on the same site as the hospice. These ladies came along, ate the cakes, sang along to the video and said that they had a thoroughly good time. Other events such as the summer fête and the inauguration of the new chaplain were more popular, suggesting that it was the past-related content of the VE Day celebrations which was particularly problematic for patients.

Patients' experiences of temporal inertia (a situation which was referred to simply and aptly by one patient as 'the waiting game') could be taken as a further indication of the loss of self many of them had experienced. Not only did patients lack a conception of a 'future self', they had also ceased to preserve a self in the present through the reconstruction and incorporation of memories from the past. Indeed, Aaronson's reflections upon time, which he sees as characterised by a past, present and future, suggest that:

> If the series is broken by removing a term or terms so that the remaining term or terms stand alone, they lose their meaning. If the present is removed *or the future and past are simultaneously eliminated a state of unbeing should result.*

(Aaronson 1972, cited in Hazan (1980: 177), emphasis added)

The material outlined above thus provides further support for the observation that a loss of mobility is associated with a loss of self through the interdependence it highlights between body, self, space and time: patients' experiences as 'body-objects' were fundamentally tied to their declining ability to negotiate space and to experience time in linear ways. Other ethnographic material can also be drawn upon to support and enhance such an analytical perspective. Ardener, for example, points to instances where practices such as foot-binding have contributed to a greater restriction of women's command of time and space. She suggests that the constriction of women's bodily movement serves as a culturally imposed mechanism for enforcing their minority (that is, 'lesser' person) status (1981: 29; see also Falk 1995: 96). Similarly, within the UK, Green points to the radical feminist critique of contemporary women's fashion (such as clothes that restrict movement and shoes that make it impossible to move fast), as serving to oppress and dominate the female gender (1991: 77).

In the instances described by Ardener and Green, the body serves as the intermediary between 'society' and the person/self, whereas in the ethnographic account here, it is the deteriorating body *per se* which imposes direct constraints upon the self. Nevertheless, in both sets of examples the relationship between bodily mobility and selfhood appears evident, particularly if one accepts Crossley's assertion that there is a compatibility between the phenomenological notion of the 'lived body' and Foucault's idea of the 'inscribed body' (1991: 99). In the case of the latter, Foucault traces the emergence of contemporary disciplinary regimes which 'construct' the modern 'Western' subject through controlling and regulating the movement of his or her body through space and time (1991: 128–9). The body thus serves as 'an intermediary' (1991: 11) through which the 'soul' or 'will' is accessed. Yet, as Crossley concludes:

> Not only can we maintain ... that inscription is only possible by virtue of an active body, we can maintain that it is only of political significance because the body is our (active) way of being-in-the-world. It is because we exist by means of embodied action that it matters how our bodies are treated and how they perform.
>
> (Crossley 1996: 114)

Transition to 'body-object': theoretical implications

The above ethnographic observations from the hospice indicate that selfhood is fundamentally tied to bodily capacity, with a loss of self occurring as patients lost the bodily ability to perform tasks for themselves. These findings thus seem to support Strathern's observation in *Dealing with Inequality* (1987) that in the modern 'West': 'From the point of view of persons, the capacity to alter the world becomes one of the prerequisites of the self-validating agent' (1987: 287). In other words, personhood depends upon agency, and agency depends upon a notion of action, of being able to 'do' and 'act' for oneself. Such a notion of agency, as Strathern highlights, stems from 'Western' understandings of the material world mediated by industrialisation,[12] which, she suggests, have led to a 'taken for granted identity between the agent as a subject and his or her actions upon the world in so far as a person's acts and work are held to belong to that person' (1987: 284). Thus ideas about industrial production – which involve the transformation of labour into products – have led 'us' to 'think about agency as the subject in subject/object relations' (1987: 286).

One can in fact take Strathern's (1987) observations to a further level of abstraction in order to understand the experiences of the high-dependency patients I encountered. It could be argued that these patients were 'taken over' by a new and powerful agent during the final stages of their illness, namely, the disease process itself, since the disease, in a sense, became the 'thing' which *caused* the patient to become immobilised.[13] It follows, then, to borrow Strathern's (1987) analytical concepts, that the patient became the 'object' in this new 'subject/object' relationship.

It is, nonetheless, important to recognise that the relationship Strathern (1987) has posited between 'Western' personhood and agency appears to involve an essentially 'disembodied' concept of the person, since the existence of a mobile and capable body – of a body which is able to 'act' – is (at most) implicitly assumed in her work.[14] And Strathern is not in isolation in this regard: as part of their wider intellectual project to 'embody' the 'subject', sociologists of the body such as Turner (1992) and Shilling and Mellor (1996) have pointed to a widespread tendency within sociological (and anthropological) theory to represent and study agency in essentially 'disembodied' ways. Their critical attention has focused, most notably, upon the work of structuration theorists such as Giddens (1979, 1984) who, they suggest, has theorised the actor as 'essentially a thinking and choosing agent, not a feeling and being agent' (Turner 1992: 87). A mind–body dualism, as Shilling and Mellor suggest, is inherent within his and other approaches, which leaves bodies somewhat problematically 'as there to be managed and moulded according to the dictates of the mind' (1996: 6). Leder, in a similar vein, has complained that, 'the notion of intentionality brings with it unnecessary philosophical baggage' because it implies 'reference to an inexistent object immanent within the subject's mind' (1990: 21). Hence there is a general plea within the work of writers such as these to incorporate a theory of the body into explorations of 'the nature of the agent in agency' (Turner 1992: 67).

The experiences of 'high-dependency' patients certainly endorse such a perspective, since they highlight something of the impossibility of retaining the status of a 'subject' and 'actor' when the physical capability to 'move' and 'act' has been lost. It is thus indeed extremely problematic to theorise agency without simultaneously according centrality to the 'active' body as the *means* of agency. Yet this leaves the challenge of making the body visible, without elevating it to an exclusive domain within academic frameworks of analysis. It is here that Merleau-Ponty's insights are particularly helpful and relevant to the project in hand. As he suggests, consciousness (and hence social being) is not so much a matter of 'I think' as of 'I can' (1962: 137). By according primacy to the latter, to the 'I can', such an analytical perspective allows agency to be theorised and understood without having to make any separation between 'mind' and 'body', 'self' and 'motion' at all.

The observations developed thus far in this chapter can, perhaps more importantly still, be used to provide a critique of much of the mainstream sociological literature on the 'performative' body. As the beginning of this chapter highlighted, most of the current literature on embodiment has focused upon, and represented, the body as the plastic or medium which is shaped by, and expresses, the will or self. What is seemingly absent in such accounts then is any obvious recognition of bodily mobility as a central part of agency. Yet, as the research outlined here has vividly revealed, this particular aspect of embodiment – the bodily ability to act – is in fact absolutely fundamental to selfhood in contexts such as modern England.

Indeed, when patients were invited to reflect on how their illness had affected their lives, it is very noteworthy that all gave primacy to the impact of their loss of bodily capacity over any other factor such as appearance (appearance being, of course, the aspect of embodiment to which most recent approaches to the body have paid the greatest attention). This phenomenon is well highlighted by Jan, who was interviewed extensively during my fieldwork in day care. At that time, Jan was ambulant, independent and able to drive herself to and from the centre. Then, she was most preoccupied with her mastectomy and the 'spoilt identity' resulting from her mutilated body (see p. 45). Nevertheless, like most day care patients, Jan was able to see herself as someone 'living with her cancer'. This situation, however, had changed substantially by the time I next met her, about nine months later. By that stage, she had been admitted to the hospice for respite care and symptom control following the spread of cancer to her bones. Jan had had to give up driving a couple of months previously. She suggested that, 'with the loss of my wheels I felt I'd lost a big part of myself'. The brittleness of her bones, coupled with accelerating weakness and lethargy, meant that she had also recently become wheelchair-bound. She poignantly suggested that it was at this stage in her deterioration that she could not see any point in continuing to live: as she pointed out, she could no longer do anything for herself.

Jan's views and experiences were shared by Doris, who had cancer of the liver. She had become very jaundiced and had substantial swelling in her lower abdomen. On one level, she clearly found her rapidly changing bodily appearance extremely distressing.[15] Nevertheless, when we started talking about the quality of her life, it became evident that she was centrally preoccupied with her increasing degree of physical dependence:

> I really don't think I've had any quality of life since I lost much of my mobility. I reckon I've only got about a quarter of the energy I used to have. Sometimes I try and do some housework, but I end up collapsed in a heap within a matter of minutes. I hate not being able to do things for myself. People are very kind and helpful, but it just isn't the same. I feel so useless. Frankly, I don't feel as if I'm living any more.

Similarly, Penny, the woman with COAD discussed above, gently reminded me that the things she missed most in life were,

> the simple things that someone like you would take for granted. ... The most important is not being able to cook my own food. I remember one time when I was in my kitchen at home and I discovered that I was too weak to pick up a saucepan. I ended up sobbing by the cooker. Another time I felt like making myself some pancakes, but I didn't have the energy to beat the eggs into the flour. ... The other thing I really miss is when I feel hot and clammy and am not able to sluice myself down. I have to ask someone else to bring me a damp flannel.

Clearly, the above ethnography and analysis call for a reappraisal of the literature on the contemporary 'Western' body. Despite the burgeoning list of texts on the body which now exist within mainstream sociology and anthropology, there is barely any recognition or reference to the fact that, in order for bodies to be 'moulded' and 'shaped' as vehicles for and expressions of the self, there have to be a minimum set of physical capacities in existence, namely those associated with the ability to act as an autonomous agent. Consequently, it could be argued that the literature has not actually succeeded in bringing the body as a material, physically experienced entity fully into social analysis. On the contrary, what appears to be examined and depicted in these particular texts is one abstraction of the body: the 'performative body'; a type of embodiment which, as we have seen, only really retains its full salience for as long as bodily mobility can be taken for granted. Beneath the seeming importance of this literally visible aspect of embodiment, the body of 'appearance, display and impression management', other aspects are equally, if not more central, to the self. Thus this study does not call for a recognition of bodily differences as such, but rather for a recognition of bodily *multiplicity*. It is only by recognising that we are embodied in multiple ways simultaneously, that one can really talk about the body as a 'lived', 'flesh and bones' entity at all.

'Objectified' bodies: carers' perspectives and experiences

So far I have focused upon patients' changing self-perceptions as their bodies weaken and deteriorate. But patients do not simply experience a shift in their self-perception from 'subject' to 'object' in isolation; in addition they are subjected to a related process of 'objectification' by those participating in their care. Carers' accounts and perspectives thus provide a further avenue for exploring the transition to 'body-objects' that high-dependency patients experience. Yet, by incorporating carers into the picture, a new but related series of themes also emerge. As we shall now see, a patient's bodily deterioration does not simply affect him or her in isolation, it may also impact upon the bodies and selves of the people involved with his or her immediate bodily care.

The 'objectification' of high-dependency patients by carers was highlighted particularly graphically in the case of Glenda, a woman with MS, admitted to the hospice for a week's respite care. Glenda's illness was extremely advanced: she was bed-bound and had lost virtually all capacity for movement from the neck downwards. Her ability to speak was severely impaired (she had to communicate by pointing her eyes towards a board with simple symbols on it). She had also lost her swallowing reflex and, consequently, had to be fed intravenously via an electronic pump dispensing liquid food directly into her stomach. When Glenda was admitted, nursing staff failed to connect her to her intravenous feeding system. The error was not noticed until the following morning.[16] When, however, nurses apologetically reported this oversight to her husband, he did not appear in the least bit bothered or upset. In fact, a little later on in the day he suggested to me that it would be no bad thing if Glenda were disconnected from her feed from time to time as it would cause her to lose weight. As he went on to point out, 'it might make it easier for me to manage her when she comes home'. In one of the staff hand-overs, the nurses expressed their admiration at the husband's ability to care for Glenda single-handed at home. On that particular day it had required four of them to lift her out of bed with a hoist so that they could give her a bath.

What this example highlights is the centrality of Glenda's 'dependent' body in the ways in which she was perceived and evaluated both by her husband and staff; a centrality that seemed to exclude any possibility of seeing Glenda as a social person.[17] For instance, none of the nurses expressed undue concern about how Glenda might have felt about not being fed. On the contrary, their apology was directed to her husband. Similarly, in her husband's evaluation, Glenda had become an 'object'; an object, furthermore, which he would find easier to 'manage' if its mass could be reduced. This shared perception of Glenda as a 'weight', rather than as a 'whole' person with a spectrum of social and emotional concerns, closely parallels the self-accounts of high-dependency patients who, as we have seen, frequently described themselves as being a 'burden'.[18]

When family members, such as Glenda's husband, reflected upon their personal experiences of caring for a patient at home, the intersubjective and intercorporeal impact of that patient's deterioration became very evident. Their comments indicated that the body of the patient became closely enmeshed with their own sense of self, particularly when the patient's deterioration and level of dependency upon them was very extreme (such patients were typically described by staff as requiring 'total' or 'hands-on' care). As the following quotes indicate, in the process of taking over and orchestrating the motions and actions of a patient's 'dependent' body, carers experienced what appeared to be a transition and transposition in their own sense of self:

> It was okay until about eight weeks ago when he was still able to look after himself and do things around the house. Then suddenly he started to get weaker and weaker. *I had to take over his jobs*, you know, things like dressing him, shaving him. ... Lifting him was a real problem. Before I knew it I was looking after him on a twenty-four hours a day basis. *I felt so trapped.* In the end I couldn't cope anymore. *It was really getting on top of me.* I'm glad he's in here, but I do feel guilty. Anyway, he's been spoken to and knows it's for the best.
>
> (Mrs B, emphasis added)

> I had to do everything for my mother when she became more unwell. Her cancer spread everywhere. She didn't want strangers [nurses] coming into her house. I had to protect her from that. I was up every night helping her onto the toilet and changing her pads ... my days were taken up feeding her, turning her [in bed]. ... Now I think about it, I don't feel as if I've been leading my own life for at least the last six months. *I've been leading someone else's; my mother's I suppose.*
>
> (Mrs F, emphasis added)

Comments such as these suggest that a patient's 'dependent' body not only dictated their own sense of self, but also the selfhood of persons caring for that body. The 'trapped' metaphor employed by Mrs B is perhaps no coincidence. It implies that her own self had become grounded in, and constrained by, the immediate physical requirements of her husband's body; her 'I can', as it were, had extended to include and enact the bodily 'tasks' of her dependent husband. Such a phenomenon can also be inferred from Mrs F's remarks: in the process of becoming the agent of her mother's bodily actions, it appears that her mother's body had become an extension of her own body and self. Hence her comment that she felt she had been leading a life other than her own; her mother's.

It was, in addition, extremely common for carers (including the two above) to speak for 'dependent' patients and to make decisions on their behalf,[19] a phenomenon which similarly indicated that the patient; the 'body-object', had become assimilated into the carer's own selfhood.[20]

> Margie was admitted yesterday. She's bed-bound and ex-
> tremely lethargic. Her daughter and son-in-law visited her
> at lunch time today and were sitting by her bed when Dr. C
> conducted his rounds. The daughter was feeding Margie,
> because she was too weak to lift a fork to her mouth her-
> self. When Dr. C came over to Margie's bed, her daughter
> asked him how much longer her mother had left to live
> [note: if Margie had chosen to do so, she was well capable
> of asking this question for herself]. He gently hinted that
> Margie probably had 'little time left'. As soon as Dr. C
> moved on to his next patient, Margie's daughter and son-
> in-law began to discuss which relatives they should con-
> tact. Margie was ignored during this conversation and
> made no effort to join in for that matter.
>
> (extract from fieldnotes)

The experiences of carers in their interactions with 'dependent' patients thus present situations wherein the self (in these interactional moments at least) is not always and necessarily singular, unified and self-contained within the parameters of an 'individuated' body. On the contrary, when one person (a carer) takes responsibility for the 'hands-on' care of another (a patient), it appears that the body of the latter becomes incorporated into the 'motoric possibilities' (Leder 1990: 163) of the former. Such a phenomenon can perhaps be most satisfactorily understood by returning to the analysis of agency developed earlier. One could argue that it is because agency, in actuality, involves a fusion of mind and body, self and action, that the body of the 'dependent' patient becomes assimilated into the 'I can' of the person who can 'act'. A new corporeal unit is thereby formed in which the selfhood of the carer is located and experienced within two bodies simultaneously (the carer's and the patient's). Agency, in a sense, resides in the location of bodily actions themselves (see below), hence the carer's self extends into the body of the 'dependent' patient she or he is tending to and moving around. Indeed it may well be for similar reasons that mothers, for example, often regard new born (and thus highly-dependent) infants as extensions of their own bodies and selves (see Grosz 1994).[21]

The material outlined above has broader theoretical implications because it can be used to destabilise the 'rhetorics of individuality' upon which many anthropological and other academic models of 'Western' personhood have typically been premised. Such a rhetoric has, for example, been drawn upon by Geertz to describe the 'Western' person as, 'a bounded, unique, more or less integrated motivational and cognitive universe, a dynamic centre of awareness, emotion, judgement and action organized into a distinctive whole and set contrastively both against other such wholes and against a social and natural background' (1984: 126). Macfarlane, likewise, describes 'English individualism' as 'the view that society is constituted of autonomous equal units, namely separate individuals and that such individuals are more important, ultimately, than any larger constituent group' (1978: 5). We have seen examples here, however, which cast doubt upon the conception that the 'Western' person is always a 'unique and indivisible unity' (La Fontaine 1985: 124), which is separate from other people and a wider social whole, 'as in our contrasting ideas about society working upon individuals and individuals shaping society' (Strathern 1988: 13).

Indeed, such an equation between body, self and personhood has already come under attack in the writings of academics such as Strathern (1988). Strathern's critical focus is not actually upon 'Western' personhood as such; rather, she is concerned to demonstrate an ethnocentrism inherent within the anthropological (and other) disciplines more generally: that anthropologists (and others) may have (wrongly) depicted 'non-Western' cultures in terms of an 'individual/society' dichotomy which, she suggests, is derived from 'Western' stereotypical understandings of personhood (1988: 13). For Strathern, such a dichotomy cannot be assumed to be universally valid, and to demonstrate this point, she uses her Melanesian study to present a somewhat different picture of sociality. Mount Hageners, she suggests, 'do not cause their own actions; they are not the authors of their own intentions' (1988: 273). In a cultural setting in which economic systems are governed by systems of gift-exchange, a person's identity, she argues, is constructed through and within transactions; identity, in a sense, inheres in the actions themselves. Thus, for Strathern's Mount Hageners at least, identity is not fixed and singular (that is, it is not the 'property' of an 'individual') and it cannot be contrastively set against a coherent, greater whole ('a society').

Strathern (1988) thus uses her Melanesian material to question one of the paradigms most central to anthropological and sociological theory: the 'individual/society' distinction. However, because her ethnographic material is drawn from a 'non-Western' context, she is not explicitly concerned with the extent to which such 'rhetorics of individuality' *actually* apply within 'Western' settings themselves. It is in this regard, then, that the study here furthers such debates.

Indeed, the observations developed in this part of the chapter suggest that no simple congruence can necessarily be drawn between rhetorical models of the 'Western' person/self (such as those contained within academic discourse) on the one hand, and the actual experiences of ordinary people on the other: rhetorics and reality would seem to rest in a somewhat uneasy partnership. Yet, as Moore's work usefully highlights, the lack of disparity between the two may actually also stem from the fact that the concept of a unified, post-Enlightenment subject itself is now out of date (1994: 55). Hence her suggestion that 'recent feminist and post-structuralist critiques of the humanist subject' (1994: 54) could be usefully be explored instead.

Certainly, the work of post-modernist writers such as Battersby (1993) and Haraway (1991) provides one possible avenue for understanding the overlapping, intersubjective experiences observed in this study. Both writers point to developments in science and technology since World War II to explain the shift away from conceptualising and experiencing the body as a 'self-contained unity' or 'bounded container' (Battersby 1993: 31) to a 'dissipative system' encompassing potentiality and flow (1993: 38). Haraway, for example, suggests that 'we are living through movement from an organic industrial society to a polymorphous information system' (1991: 161), in which communications technologies and biotechnologies are 'the crucial tools recrafting our bodies' (1991: 164). The changing 'social relationships of science and technology', she suggests, have led to a blurring of machine and organism such that 'mind, body, and tool are on very intimate terms' (1991: 165).[22] Such a phenomenon, as she further observes, throws into question whether 'our bodies end at the skin' (1991: 178); in other words, the self and subjectivity may extend beyond the parameters of an 'individuated' body (Stone 1995: 395; Downey 1995: 364). Battersby, in a similar vein, suggests that within the new scientific, mathematical and topographical models that have superseded hylomorphism:

there is no fundamental difference between states and forms: forms simply are structurally stable moments within the evolution of a system (or space). Indeed, for a new form to emerge on this model the entire space or system is itself subject to transformation or distortion from exterior spaces or systems. We are dealing here with open dissipative systems and with leaks of energy into and out of the system.

(Battersby 1993: 35)[23]

The new metaphysics entailed by such topological models have thus led to a conception of self which is not necessarily located inside the body (1993: 32); on the contrary, the concept of 'bodily containment' must itself be questioned (1993: 36). As Battersby suggests: 'The boundary of my body should rather be thought of as an event-horizon, in which one form (myself) meets its potentiality for transforming itself into another form or forms' (ibid.). The self can thus be conceived of as a 'dissipative system' which can encompass other systems, bodies and selves (ibid.); agency, as Battersby suggests, needs to be theorised 'in terms of patterns of potentiality and flow' (1993: 38).

Academics such as Battersby and Haraway thus relate fluid and overlapping notions of the self to newly emerging cultural factors. It would, nonetheless, be unwise to posit too sharp a distinction between conceptions and experiences of selfhood prior to, and since, the scientific and technological developments they highlight, for much the same reasons as 'West/Rest' distinctions are too generalising and polarised (see, for example, Said 1991). Indeed, one major shortcoming of Haraway's and Battersby's approaches is that they do not explicitly address generational issues: it is extremely likely that the 'social relationships of science and technology' that they explore have impacted more fundamentally upon junior than senior generations. It is likely, therefore, that post-modern studies of the types outlined above can provide little more than partial explanations for the 'fluid' nature of the self highlighted in patient–carer interactions.

Whether or not one accepts arguments such as Haraway's in their entirety, an interesting parallel can be drawn between my observation that the body of a dependent patient becomes merged with the self of a carer when she or he takes on responsibility for that patient's 'hands-on' care, and her observation that machines and other prosthetic devices can become 'intimate components, friendly selves' (1991: 178). In much the same way as carers assimilate a patient's body into their own self when they become the agent of his or her body tasks, prosthetic devices assisting mobility (such as a walking stick) can become an extrapolation and extension of that particular person/self. It is very significant that, when one of the patients I encountered in day care became too weak to drive his own car, he likened the experience to losing his right arm. Both a carer and a prosthesis become merged with a patient's body, because what both have in common is that they constitute the source and/or means of that patient's bodily mobility.

And it is because objects and instruments which facilitate mobility can become a part of a patient's self that situations do occur in which those with 'high-dependency' needs can preserve or reconstitute the self through the use and assimilation of prosthetic devices: Stephen Hawking being a notable case in point (see Stone 1995). Seymour (1998), for example, has studied the long-term rehabilitation of men and women who, following damage to the spinal cord, became paraplegic or quadriplegic. As her study reveals, learning to use a wheelchair and other devices (and thus re-acquiring the ability to act without assistance from others) is a central means by which those suffering from bodily impairment can 'remake' not only their bodies but also their selves.[24] Yet, because rehabilitation requires comparatively long periods of time such a phenomenon did not, and indeed could not, occur amongst many of the hospice patients with whom I worked. These patients often experienced a very rapid deterioration in their bodily capabilities: there was, quite simply, insufficient time for adjustments to be made before further degeneration or death occurred.

The 'dying' patient and the 'loss' of the person

As patients approached death, it thus became increasingly difficult for them to perform those tasks, and enter into those social interactions, that allowed them to be considered persons. It is not surprising, therefore, that there came a stage in most patients' deterioration at which their visitors' behaviour and attitude towards them indicated that, in their perception, the person had already 'gone'. Hospice staff, for example, often made a clear distinction between patients who were 'dying' and those who were not. The fact that such a boundary was drawn suggests that, in their perception, 'dying' denoted a significant, and in most cases irreversible, 'status passage' (Glaser and Strauss 1971). Different members of the multi-disciplinary team's definitions of 'dying' were fairly consistent, as can be seen from the responses I received when I asked staff to suggest the criteria used to classify a patient as dying:

When the patient slips into a coma.

(nurse)

When the body starts to shut down physically and the patient switches off mentally.

(occupational therapist)

When the patient drifts into a coma. More specifically, I suppose, when they cease to be able to communicate and have become unaware of their environment.

(chaplain)

When the level of dependency combined with the degree of physical weakness is such that the patient can do nothing for themselves. Normally the patient has slipped into a coma or a semi-coma by this stage.

(doctor)

What all these definitions encompass is the idea that dying involves a state of total physical dependency, together with a loss of awareness of oneself and one's environment. Indeed, no distinction needs to be made here between 'physical' and 'mental' criteria because dying patients lack bodily autonomy and outward displays of sentience simultaneously: one could argue that such patients constitute 'body-objects' in the most extreme form.

The hospice doctor quoted above went on to suggest that she was sympathetic to the argument for euthanasia when a patient had reached this stage in his/her deterioration, 'particularly if their condition drags on in this liminal state for days, as sometimes happens'.[25] Her inference was that the person/self had already gone. Such a view also appeared to be shared by the majority of family and friends who made visits to the hospice. I frequently observed that their behaviour and attitude towards a patient changed notably once that patient was judged to be dying. Visitors commonly used phrases such as 'not the same person', 'not herself', or more commonly still, 'too far gone' and 'already left' when they talked about a dying patient. The regular use of metaphors pertaining to space and time indicates carers' perceptions that the person had already 'gone' leaving an empty body. Visitors, furthermore, often expressed a high degree of ambivalence about whether it was helpful to a comatose patient, or even appropriate, to continue to spend time with them. Interestingly, they rarely suggested that this ambivalence stemmed from a fear or anxiety about seeing the patient die. It thus does not seem, as the work of writers such as Gorer (1965) and Ariès (1981) suggests, that it was the taboo nature of death *per se* which was at issue. On the contrary, visitors' mixed feelings appeared to stem from their perception that their relative or friend had already 'departed'. One woman, for instance, left the hospice after her mother had slipped into a coma, explaining that, 'I just can't see any point in being here. She doesn't know who I am. ... I feel as if she's already dead.' Her mother's physical death did not actually occur for a further thirty-six or so hours. Other relatives and friends suggested that they did not want to visit patients once they were dying because they wished to remember them 'as they were'. This perspective again implies that a dying patient had ceased to be the person visitors once knew.

On occasions when a patient's death was particularly drawn out (sometimes patients could remain comatose for days or even weeks), it was common for relatives to suggest that 'it will be one big relief when the whole thing's over with', even if the patient looked peaceful and did not appear to be suffering. Such a comment would frequently be followed by an expression of guilt and embarrassment that the carer could suggest 'such a terrible thing'. Other visitors, however, were less inhibited in expressing their views. After one patient, Colin, had been in a coma for two days, his wife and daughter approached the Senior Registrar and suggested the following: 'Why don't you give him a big injection and get the whole bloody thing over and done with.'

As the above observations highlight, once a patient had slipped into a coma, visitors often appeared to make a distinction between the cessation of the person and the patient's physical cessation, which could occur hours, or sometimes days, afterwards. The comment of Colin's relatives, in particular, indicates a desire for a patient's physical death to be brought forward to concur more closely with the demise of his or her personhood. Findings such as these have also been echoed by researchers working in different settings. Lock, for example, in her study of brain death and organ transplantation, observes that newspaper and television accounts regularly report that patients who have been declared 'brain dead' later 'die' when life-support measures are removed, and, furthermore, health professionals regularly use terminology that implies that such patients 'die twice' (1996: 220). The idea that 'life may go on after the person has died' (Bartlett and Younger 1988: 211) has also been recognised in various sociological, ethical and media debates surrounding the moral and legal status of patients in persistent vegetative states (PVS). Such debates have focused primarily upon the question of whether PVS patients are persons 'to whom continued medical treatment is due' (Zaner 1988: vii) or if, in fact, the person has 'gone', 'leaving a residual body that continues to respire spontaneously because of the presence of an intact brain stem' (ibid.; see also White 1988: 104; Lamb 1990: 44).

A survey of the research literature on Alzheimer's disease also allows some points of similarity and of departure to be drawn. Alzheimer's is typically described as a disease that robs the victim of their mind (Fontana and Smith (1989) because it causes a 'progressive and usually irreversible deterioration of mental capacities' (Jenkins and Price 1996: 84). This situation, as Downs observes, often leads to the conception that patients suffering from Alzheimer's disease (and other forms of dementia) experience, 'a steady erosion of personality and identity' to a stage where 'no person' remains (1997: 597). Herskovits, in a similar vein, points to 'the debased personhood implicit in the current Alzheimer's construct' (1995: 148). Such a phenomenon, she suggests, is exemplified in the metaphors and images of Alzheimer's disease as 'a funeral without an end', 'the loss of self', and the 'death before death' (ibid.). Orona likewise observes in her interviews with carers of family members with Alzheimer's disease that, by the time they had decided to have a patient placed in long-term institutional care, carers felt that, 'the person they had once known as husband, mother or wife, was "gone". They were institutionalising "strangers". The person who they had once known had changed to the point of being dead' (1990: 1249).

Yet, what would seemingly distinguish patients with Alzheimer's disease and other forms of dementia from those in a coma or a PVS is the retention of their bodily capabilities. I emphasise the word *seemingly* here because academics who have conducted research amongst patients with Alzheimer's disease and their families rarely point to, or address, the fact that many of these patients also suffer from some degree of bodily impairment. Dementing illnesses occur most commonly amongst the older people (especially those in their eighties and nineties) who are thus also likely to be suffering from a number of chronic and debilitating *bodily* conditions (for example, osteoporosis and arthritis). In the later stages of its progression, furthermore, the effects of Alzheimer's disease may become manifest in embodied ways: cognitive impairment may, for instance, lead to disorientation and, in some instances, to a loss of ability to control bowel and bladder functions. As we shall see in the following chapter, a loss of continence, like a loss of bodily mobility, may also have an absolutely 'non-negotiable' impact upon a patient's self.

Whilst it is thus somewhat misleading to represent, and to study, the loss of self experienced amongst Alzheimer's patients as simply a phenomenon stemming from 'mental' degeneration, the literature outlined above does open up a new avenue of enquiry which has not, as yet, been considered extensively in this book. Since Alzheimer's patients appear to experience an 'inexorable dissolution of self' (Cohen and Eisdorfer 1986: 22) without necessarily reaching a stage at which they require 'total bodily care', it seems unwise to posit a straightforward and exclusive equation between a 'loss of self' and a loss of 'I can'. It appears that other factors also require consideration. It is in this respect that Orona's study provides us with some further interesting insights. According to Orona's observations, the person with Alzheimer's was considered to be 'gone' at the stage when they ceased to be able to recognise their carers, and thus to engage in interactions with them, such that 'each member *reciprocally* participates in the maintenance and transformation of the other's identity' (1990: 1251, original emphasis). Carers, she suggests, had thus lost a person who could validate their own past experience and provide the promise of such validation in the future (1990: 1254). Such a situation, as she further notes, caused carers to feel that they had also lost remnants of their own sense of self (1990: 1255). I shall return to the central part that interpersonal relationships also play in formations (and losses) of self in Chapter 5, where I focus specifically upon these exterior aspects of selfhood.

The dying patient and the 'hospice body'

As I highlighted in Chapter 1, hospice care, according to its formal objectives, set itself the goal of sustaining a patient's person/self to the moment of physical death, thereby enabling patients to 'live until they die'. As we have seen in this chapter, however, such an objective is often not realisable in practice, because hospice professionals have to contend with what I have termed 'the bodily realities of dying', that is, the fundamental impact that a patient's bodily deterioration may have upon his or her self. Thus, in the case of dying patients in particular, hospices are often left caring for a body, not a person. Yet, as I now examine, in supporting another of its central ideological tenets – an open confrontation with death – hospice care appears, to some extent, to reinforce this reduction of the dying patient to the status of a body.

The modern hospice movement, as I examined in Chapter 1, emerged largely in response to the disillusionment of certain medical professionals with the care of dying patients in hospitals. The pioneers of the movement argued that the hiding away of death and dying in institutions has resulted in these phenomena becoming invisible to most members of society; a situation which has supposedly led to these phenomena being surrounded by unnecessary taboos. They therefore advocated an open confrontation with death, and it is this philosophy which continues to underlie the practice of keeping dying patients in communal wards in full view of other patients. Such openness, however, contrasts with the sequestration of the 'dirty work' performed by nurses (such as washing a patient and helping them onto a commode), which, as Lawler observes, occurs 'behind closed doors or behind screens' (1991: 46). In these latter instances, privacy is deemed as both appropriate and necessary in order to maintain a patient's dignity (ibid.; see also Elias 1994).

What is particularly interesting and relevant about this practice of 'public dying' is the extent to which it appeared to be done for the benefit of other hospice patients. Such a situation became very apparent in the context of a staff case conference set up to explore the ethics of keeping dying patients in wards, which was held shortly after my fieldwork began. During this meeting, staff pointed to a number of positive effects such a practice could have upon other patients present in the ward. As several participants pointed out, a number of patients admitted to the hospice had never witnessed a death firsthand and, consequently, were anxious to know what their own deaths would be like. Patients, could thus find it 'very comforting to watch another patient drift off peacefully beside them' (Nina, nurse). The staff's impressions and views also find support in two recent psychological studies (one of which was actually circulated and discussed during the meeting) that have examined the impact of patient deaths on other patients in the same hospice ward (Honeybun *et al.* 1992; Payne *et al.* 1996). Both studies found that patients who had witnessed the death of another patient were significantly less depressed than those who had not.[26]

In the case conference, staff members also pointed to the potential distress which could be caused to patients if those judged to be dying were moved out of the ward. Their rationale was as follows:

> It would make them [the other patients] think death is something to be frightened of, something we have to protect them from. If we move a dying patient, it makes the others scared. They want to know why we've taken them away.
>
> (Carrie, nurse)

What was notable by its absence from the meeting, however, was any explicit consideration of the preferences of dying patients themselves. Part of the reason for this omission may well have stemmed from the difficulty, many would say impossibility, of actually accessing the views of 'silent' patients (see Gadow 1989). Yet, the absence/omission also indicates a more fundamental, underlying issue: dying patients were not being accorded the same rights and interests (such as the right to privacy) as the other patients and participants within the hospice.[27] One might be inclined, therefore, to understand the hospice movement's advocacy of an open confrontation with death in terms of an ethic which is primarily utilitarian in nature; an ethic which both reflects and reinforces that status of a dying patient as being that of a residual body.[28] Indeed, Lawler has suggested that: 'When patients are dying ... the patient relinquishes responsibility for body care and body functions to the nurse and "hands over" the body' (1991: 183). It is tempting, however, to modify her terminology and its associated ramifications. Rather than seeing the patient as 'handing over' his or her body (which would imply choice and an act of authorship), it could be argued that hospice care in fact 'takes over' that body. In so doing, hospice care, it seems, converts the patient's body into a 'docile body' which is 'subjected and used' (Foucault 1991: 136) to 'perform ceremonies, to emit signs' (1991: 25). The dying patient's body, as I have indicated, becomes a body on 'display', a 'hospice body' located in communal space to enact the ideology of an open confrontation with death. Such an analytical perspective can also be used to provide new insights into practices such as sedating patients when they become very confused or distressed.

As I indicated earlier, the modern hospice movement's open confrontation with death is premised upon a model of a 'good death'. A 'good death', as Ariès has argued, relates to an 'acceptable' way of dying, which is itself culturally and historically variable (1974, 1981). Within the hospice where I conducted fieldwork, a good death was considered by staff to be one in which the patient 'drifted off peacefully', which, in practice, meant that the patient died free of pain and any apparent distress. In interviews with hospice nurses (McNamara et al. 1994) and also with patients (Payne et al. 1996) it was similarly found that primacy was given to patients looking 'peaceful', 'dying with dignity', 'quietly' and 'free of pain' in perceptions of characteristics constituting a 'good' hospice death. As McNamara et al. further point out, however, whilst a 'good death' is something staff 'implicitly work towards', it is 'not always readily attainable' (1994: 1504). This was indeed so in the hospice in which I worked. Patients' pain could not always be controlled (especially in the case of those dying of lung cancer), and a significant proportion also became very distressed, agitated and confused prior to their deaths. Staff pointed to a condition called 'terminal restlessness', which involved patients drifting in and out of consciousness and exhibiting what they termed 'psychotic' behaviour.[29] This condition sometimes resulted in the patient becoming aggressive, shouting out, and accusing staff (and sometimes other patients) of deliberately trying to kill them.

In some cases, staff moved the patient into a side room in order to maintain what Fagerhaugh and Strauss (1977) have called the 'sentimental order' in the ward. Yet removal was often not a viable strategy because of the lack of availability of single rooms within the building. Therefore, in a number of instances staff adopted a different strategy: namely to sedate a patient heavily, thereby rendering him or her 'docile'.

> Audrey became very agitated this morning. She occasionally woke up from her semi-comatose state to discover that her legs were paralysed: 'I can't move my legs! I can't move my legs! what have you done to me? ... Help me! Help me!' Audrey demanded that the staff ring her husband and son and ask them to come in. By the time they arrived, she had

become more agitated and confused. Periodically she would scream and shout out, accusing her family and staff of making her into a 'cripple'. The other patients on the ward seemed similarly distressed and upset. Senior medical staff took her husband and son on one side and, following a brief discussion, a decision was made to sedate her. Her husband agreed that he would rather see Audrey looking 'peaceful and comfortable' than 'distressed'. Audrey was connected to a syringe pump driver which provided her with a continuous dose of sedatives. She remained unconscious until she died two days later.

(extract from fieldnotes)

In this and other similar instances, staff emphasised that their reason for sedating patients was so that they 'looked peaceful'. Their comments thus concur with the formal rhetoric of hospice care which contends that patients are sedated to 'alleviate' their 'distress' and 'enable them to rest peacefully' (National Council for Hospice and Specialist Palliative Care Services 1993: 8), a rhetoric which in and of itself appears to be relatively altruistic and benign. Yet, as Fagerhaugh and Strauss have pointed out, sedation puts 'the patient into a living sleep with drugs', and thus constitutes an imposed 'social death' (1977: 162). In removing a patient's sentience through sedation the last vestiges of their personhood are also erased; aspects of person and self which involve patients' ability to 'act', choose and make decisions for themselves. It seems important, therefore, to explore the extent to which such a practice is actually done for the benefit of the dying patient him or herself. Impromptu remarks made by staff suggest an alternative perspective. One hospice nurse, for example, commented that, 'for all we know patients might prefer to go out shouting and screaming'. Another nurse expressed her underlying qualms that sometimes patients were sedated,

> more for our benefit, and for the benefit of the family and the other patients. The bottom line is that people don't want to see someone going out looking so upset and distressed. It makes our job so much more stressful and difficult.

It thus appears that the practice of sedation is not grounded solely in an ethics of beneficence; that is, in a 'commitment to promoting only the individual patient's best interest' (Gadow 1989: 536), if indeed such interest can ever be satisfactorily ascertained (Gadow 1989: 537). It actually requires little imagination to argue that sedation was in fact performed primarily to reinforce the hospice's ideology of a good death, particularly in view of the observation developed earlier, that such an ideology requires the location of 'docile bodies' within communal space.[30]

Other patients in the hospice made active and explicit requests for sedation when their suffering became very extreme, and it is to these patients, in particular, that this study shall now turn. Heavy sedation does not kill patients,[31] but, as we have seen, it can remove the last remnants of their personhood, transforming them into 'body-objects'. Under what conditions patients sought to end their suffering in this way, and what, in fact, constituted 'suffering' for dying patients, is examined further in the next two chapters, where I take a further look at the process of dying in the hospice, and particularly at the centrality of bodily unboundedness in hospice deaths.

4

INPATIENT HOSPICE CARE

The sequestration of the unbounded body and 'dirty dying'

Introduction

The hospice in which I conducted fieldwork underwent some major changes both before and during the ten-month period of study. As described in earlier chapters, the hospice was originally a twenty-five bed unit. Six beds were cut about a year before I started fieldwork, and a further three two months into the study. In both cases, bed cutbacks resulted from the decision of the local Health Commission (the 'purchasers') to allocate a larger proportion of its palliative care budget to primary care services. This shift reflected broader trends in care for the terminally ill. As I indicated in Chapter 1, during the past decade or so there has been a noticeable transition away from hospitals and other institutions as the site for death and dying in the UK. A number of studies suggest that, if given a choice, the majority of terminally ill patients would prefer to be cared for and die in their own homes rather than in the sanitised and impersonal environment of the hospital (see, for example, Thorpe 1993; Townsend *et al.* 1990; Dunlop *et al.* 1989). Whilst a lot of contention and debate surrounds this issue (some scholars argue, for instance, that the desirability of a home death is a form of rhetoric congenial to policy makers and planners, promoted by them because it is a more cost-effective form of care[1] (Holmes 1995; Neale 1993; Parker 1990)), it remains the case that a progressive shift is occurring towards the care of patients with advanced and terminal illnesses in 'the community'. Hence, as Lunt has observed in his overview of terminal cancer care services in Great Britain, a switch in emphasis is taking place at the policy and planning level from the establishment and support of hospice inpatient units to the financing of home care services (1985: 753; see also Taylor 1983; Eve *et al.* 1997: 42).

The permanent closure of beds had a direct impact upon the types of patient admitted to the hospice. Bed shortages necessitated a review of the hospice's admissions policy and, as a consequence, a decision was made to reduce the number of respite admissions substantially. By the end of my fieldwork, admissions for non-cancer respite patients were stopped altogether. Both the hospice doctors and the NHS managers argued that the young chronically sick were 'constipating the service', by 'blocking beds' and 'draining scarce nursing time and resources' away from more 'pressing' and 'deserving' cases. Priority was given to patients exhibiting particularly distressing bodily symptoms, especially during the terminal phase of their illness. Furthermore, owing to the increased pressure to free beds, the hospice also encouraged the earliest possible discharge for all its patients. Whenever it was viable, patients were returned to their homes after a one-week or two-week stay in the hospice (indeed, some patients were discharged home to die). Thus, as I examine below, the patients who were most likely to remain within the hospice on a longer-term basis were those who had escalating symptoms which could not be successfully treated or controlled by medical staff, and who were therefore deemed inappropriate for home-based care.

The commonly accepted argument that patients are sequestered within hospices because of the taboo nature of death and dying in contemporary 'Western' societies (Mellor 1993) seems, therefore, untenable: a significant proportion of patients are now cared for and do die at home. Certainly, in the part of England where I conducted fieldwork approximately one-third of all cancer deaths occurred at home, with the remaining two-thirds being divided roughly equally between the hospice and the hospital. It was not dying as such but rather specific kinds of demise that were to be found within the hospice. Within the developing climate of community care, the hospice was progressively able only to cater for those patients who could not be looked after within 'the community', because 'the community' could not accommodate them either practically or symbolically. As the following ethnography and analysis will highlight, it is important to focus upon the body of the patient, and the disease processes taking place within it and upon its surfaces, in order to understand why some patients were contained within the bounded space of the hospice whereas others were not. I argue that contemporary inpatient hospices, such as the one observed during my fieldwork, are increasingly becoming enclaves in which a particular type of bodily deterioration and decay is set apart from mainstream society. In so doing, hospices and other similar institutions enable certain ideas about 'living', personhood and the physically bounded body to be symbolically enforced and maintained.

This chapter will thus be concerned with a special case of loss of bodily autonomy: the loss of control of the body's physical boundaries. The physically bounded body, as we shall see, is another aspect of embodiment which is central to selfhood in modern English contexts; a feature of person and self which, again, only becomes evident as such after it has been lost.

I begin here with an extended case study of a patient named Annie. In some respects the following example is remarkable because her death was considered by staff to be one of the most distressing that occurred within the hospice during the period of my fieldwork. Nevertheless, it provides a useful starting point because Annie's experience encompasses a number of features shared entirely or in part by the majority of patients who, at the time of my research, were receiving care within the hospice.

Case study – Annie

Annie was 67 when she was first admitted to the hospice on 12 April 1995. Prior to her admission, she had been living at home with her retired husband and recently divorced son. She also had a married daughter living locally.

Annie had been diagnosed as having cancer of the cervix in April 1994. Following surgery and post-operative radiotherapy it was believed that she had made a full recovery. However, in February 1995 a smear test revealed a large recurrence which was subsequently found to have spread to her pelvic wall. Annie was informed by her doctor that there was little further that could be done for her because her cancer was too far advanced. She was referred to a Macmillan nurse for palliative care in March.

Initially, she managed at home with regular medical and emotional support from her District and Macmillan nurses. At this stage, her greatest problem stemmed from the development of severe oedema in both of her legs which had caused her to become bed-bound.[2] She found it difficult to relinquish her duties as 'housewife' to her husband and son, and was still trying to manage the household from her bed.

Annie's mobility improved a little after she received lymphoedema treatment at home. She became sufficiently ambulant to take herself independently to the bathroom, but she remained largely confined to bed. With the encouragement and support of her Macmillan nurse, she began to tie up some of her 'loose ends', such as writing a will. Her nurse reported that Annie and her family were 'terrified' about what the future held in store for them.

At the beginning of April, Annie's condition began to deteriorate. She developed a recto-vaginal fistula, which meant that her urine and faeces started coming out through the same passageway. Problems of faecal leakage precipitated her admission to the hospice for symptom control.

Originally Annie had been very anxious about the possibility of being admitted to the hospice. As she explained about one week into her stay: 'Initially I didn't want to come in here because I didn't think I'd get out again.' In fact, when recurrence of cancer was first diagnosed, she made her family promise that they would do everything possible to enable her to stay at home. It is highly relevant, therefore, that it was Annie herself who finally pressed for an admission. One reason she gave for doing so was her concern about how exhausted her husband had become; 'I could see him crumbling in front of me'. Yet the other reason she presented seemed even more significant: Annie said she did not have enough privacy at home to attend to her personal hygiene. She had become semi-incontinent and was also suffering from periodic bouts of diarrhoea, which she found deeply distressing and embarrassing. She did not want her family to witness her bodily degradation first hand.

Following her admission to the hospice, Annie was placed in one of the wards. Initially, she was sufficiently mobile to take herself independently to the toilet and bathroom, and she remained stubbornly 'self-caring' even though she had to spend up to an hour cleaning herself after using the toilet. Whilst, superficially, she seemed bright and cheerful, night staff reported a very different picture: Annie was frequently heard sobbing quietly to herself whilst locked inside the toilet.

About ten days into her admission, Annie deteriorated further. Her fistula enlarged substantially and, as a result, every time she attempted to get out of bed and stand up, diarrhoea and urine would pour straight out of her body. Consequently, she had to start using a commode in the ward rather than walking to the toilet. A day or so later, she also contracted a bladder infection which caused her urine to develop a very offensive smell.

It was around this time that Annie's bodily degradation began to have a significant impact upon the hospice as a whole. Whenever she used the commode in the ward, the smell would penetrate right through the building to the main entrance. Staff burnt aromatherapy oils around her bed, but, generally, these did little to mask the odour. The other patients complained that sometimes the smell made them want to vomit.

Annie became increasingly anxious about the possibility of being discharged home. She felt she had lost all her dignity. She also stressed that there would be insufficient privacy at home to mask the smell and her degradation from her family. At the multidisciplinary team meeting to discuss her case, the Senior Consultant argued that it would be 'cruel and futile' to press for a discharge. None of the other members of staff challenged his decision in spite of the economic pressures to free her bed. There was no further talk of discharge and Annie and her family were promised that she could remain in the hospice until she died.

Throughout the rest of the month, Annie continued to deteriorate. She 'rotted away below', as the nurses put it, and lost all control over her bowel and bladder functions. As a consequence, she suffered from continuous bouts of incontinence. It proved impossible to keep her clean and her sheets fresh. On several occasions when the nurses came to attend to her, they found her covered to her shoulders in her own urine and excreta.

By this stage, the smell resulting from her incontinence had become a perpetual problem, and staff became increasingly concerned about the impact Annie's bodily deterioration was having upon the other patients in her ward. They suggested that she might prefer the privacy of a side room, but Annie remained adamant that she wanted to 'stay with the ladies'. Like a number of the other working-class patients I encountered in the hospice, she was worried that she would feel lonely if placed in a room on her own (see Chapter 5). She also appeared to have become more or less oblivious to her own smell: whilst she was lucid on some occasions, she was also suffering from increased bouts of tiredness and confusion.

Since Annie had made it clear that she did not want to be moved to a side room, staff were left with the problem of what to do with the other patients in her ward. Whilst none of the other patients were actually moved out of the ward because of Annie's presence, I did observe that when a patient died or was discharged their bed was not refilled. In fact, by the time I became closely involved with Annie's case (which was about three weeks into her stay in the hospice), only two other women remained in her ward. Paula had brain secondaries and had been admitted to the hospice for terminal care. She remained uncommunicative and unaware of her environment until she died. Doris, however, was fully lucid and became deeply upset by Annie's deterioration: she requested her own discharge, pointing to 'the terrible smell' and Annie's distress as the main precipitating factors. She also made it very clear that under no circumstances did she ever want to return to the hospice, and needed a lot of reassurance that her own death was unlikely to be as undignified and distressing as Annie's.

The morning that Doris was discharged, Annie became very tearful and afraid. I was asked by one of the senior nurses to go and sit with her until her husband and the hospice chaplain arrived. Annie told me that she was convinced that she was being punished for all the wrongs in her life; she suggested that she must have committed some terrible sin in the past for God to inflict such a cruel 'exit' upon her. She was also upset that her husband had written her a romantic card the previous day telling her how much he loved her. She wanted to know why he was saying this to her now, when he had never done so in the past. She complained of feeling worthless and the object of other people's pity.

As the morning went on, Annie became increasingly agitated and afraid. Her diarrhoea escalated, and at lunch time she asked to be sedated. Senior medical staff fulfilled her request after she repeated it several further times. This was the last time I spoke to her: she remained heavily sedated and unconscious until she died approximately two weeks later.

The day after Annie was first sedated, Paula, the other woman remaining in her ward, died. Once Paula's body had been removed from the ward, staff felt they had no option but to move Annie to a side room. They approached her family and explained that they could not really admit any patients to Annie's ward because of the smell. The family readily gave their consent for Annie to be moved. Both her husband and son expressed their embarrassment that she had been 'stinking out' the ward for so long.

Once Annie had been settled into her side room, visits from her family dropped off rapidly. They could not see any point, they said, in keeping a vigil around her bed when she was almost certainly oblivious to their presence. It is also noteworthy that the stench of incontinence and decaying flesh was considerably stronger in the side room than it had been in the ward.

In the final days of her life, staff kept Annie comfortable by increasing her doses of diamorphine. She did not actually die until the early hours of 16 May, which was approximately six weeks after she was first admitted to the hospice. None of her family was present at the time of her death.

Outside:inside / boundedness:unboundedness – inpatient hospice care and the unbounded body

Annie's case will be referred to at various points in this chapter because of the rich and complex issues it brings to the fore. However, the one theme I want to focus upon at this stage concerns the way in which the development and spread of her cervical cancer affected her body. One of the main factors which precipitated Annie's admission to the hospice for symptom control was the development of a fistula which resulted in faecal leakage. As the fistula enlarged, she ceased to have any control over her bowel and bladder functions. Because the management of the effects of this breakdown of bodily control ceased to be effective, all plans for a discharge were abandoned.

In this respect, Annie's case was far from atypical: during the course of my fieldwork, the most common reason for a patient to be admitted to the hospice was for 'symptom control', a phenomenon which became especially marked after the number of beds were cut. In a study conducted to identify the factors influencing the admission of patients to St Christopher's hospice in London, Woodhall similarly found that 'the major cause of admission is either "poor symptom control" or "good to fairly good symptom control" which subsequently fails' (1986: 32; see also Eve *et al.* 1997). Significantly, most symptoms requiring 'control' appeared to share a distinctive feature in common: they were associated with, or caused, a rupturing and breakdown of the surfaces of a patient's body. As a consequence, fluids and matter normally contained within the body were leaked and emitted to the outside, often in an uncontrolled and *ad hoc* fashion. Staff often employed metaphors such as 'falling apart at the seams' when referring to patients who were 'rotting inside' and 'being eaten away by their cancer'. Patients requiring symptom control thus had bodies which I will term here as 'unbounded', meaning the literal erosion of the patient's physical boundaries.

Symptom control encompassed a wide range of bodily ailments and their side-effects. Amongst the most common were incontinence of urine and faeces; uncontrolled vomiting (including faecal vomit); fungating tumours (the rotting away of a tumour site on the surface of the skin); and weeping limbs which resulted from the development of gross oedema in a patient's legs and/or arms (the limbs would swell to such an extent that the skin burst and lymph fluid continuously seeped out).

Other symptoms, though less common, were equally significant. For example, several emergency admissions occurred after a patient started coughing up large amounts of blood at home. In another instance a patient, Tony, was admitted after he developed a facial tumour. Apart from causing a gross distortion of his features (Tony's left eye was gradually being pushed sideways and out of its socket), the expanding tumour was also causing the arteries in his nasal area to rupture. As a result, he suffered from continuous nose bleeds, and had to have a bolus of cloth permanently attached beneath his nose to absorb the frequent outpourings of blood and mucus. The hospice's doctors predicted that Tony's death could be caused at any time by a 'catastrophic nose bleed' and for this reason were very reluctant to consider a discharge. Similarly, Marie developed a large tumour in her groin area. During her seven-week stay in the hospice, it swelled to the size of a rugby ball. On a number of occasions the tumour site partially ruptured, causing blood to spurt out onto the nurses attending to her. Again, staff believed Marie was 'living with a time bomb' as her swelling could burst at any time and cause her to bleed to death.

On a number of occasions, patients' symptoms were successfully treated or controlled by medical staff, and the boundedness of their bodies was thus reinstated. For example, several patients were admitted with incontinence of urine, and were able to return home once they had been catheterised. Other symptoms, such as violent and repeated vomiting and diarrhoea, could often be treated through changes in diet and medication, and weeping limbs and fungating tumours through the application of dressings and bandages. Having had their bodies successfully 'rebounded', it was then possible, and indeed common, for patients to be discharged. In this respect the hospice could be understood as a mediator between the unbounded and the bounded body, with patients being moved into the hospice when the surfaces of their bodies ruptured and broke down, and moved out again when their bodily boundedness and integrity were subsequently restored.

A number of patients, however, like Annie, had symptoms which escalated following their admission to the hospice and, as a consequence, the boundedness of their bodies was impossible to reinstate. These patients, who will form the focus of the following ethnography and discussions, were the ones most likely to remain within the hospice until they died. What is striking about this subgroup of patients is that many appeared to experience a loss of self once their bodies became severely and irreversibly unbounded, in spite of the fact that they often retained their sentience and capacity for mobility.

Annie was one of several patients admitted with recto-vaginal fistulas during my fieldwork. Another woman, Deborah, experienced a similar trajectory of deterioration and decline. She was originally admitted for a blood transfusion but the developing fistula, coupled with periodic bouts of confusion (possibly caused by the spread of cancer to her brain), kept her in the hospice until she died.

Staff considered Deborah a very difficult patient to look after. One night, for example, members of the nursing team were kept occupied for several hours after she disappeared from her side room. She was eventually found in the staff toilets totally covered in excreta. The walls and floor of the toilet were also splattered with her faeces. Deborah had by then recovered from her temporarily confused state and was deeply upset and embarrassed. After this incident, staff decided to move her into one of the wards so that it would be easier to keep an eye on her. Around this time, Deborah's deterioration began to escalate and her incontinence became more or less continuous. Members of the nursing staff found it necessary to change her pads at least four times at night.

When Deborah's bodily deterioration escalated, I noticed that she suddenly became much more withdrawn. After she had been in the ward for a couple of days, she started asking for the curtains to be drawn around her bed to give her more privacy. A day or so later, she stopped talking altogether, unless it was really necessary (to ask for the commode for example), even when her family and other visitors were present. She also refused all food and drink. Deborah spent the remaining ten days of her life either sleeping or staring blankly into space. Staff also became aware of this 'strange' behaviour. One of the hospice doctors concluded that, 'for all intents and purposes, she [had] shut herself off in a frustrated and irreversible silence'. Deborah was moved back into a side room and died there a couple of days later.

130

I spoke to Deborah's daughter about a month after she had died and she reflected very frankly and openly upon her mother's death. She felt she had actually said her 'good-byes' to Deborah about a week before she died (i.e. around the time her mother had become very withdrawn): 'After that she really wasn't there anymore ... she wasn't my mother.'

In Deborah's case, then, it appears that she 'disengaged' and 'switched off' prior to her physical cessation. Such an experience seemed to be shared by a number of patients with unbounded bodies, especially those whose bodily unboundedness became very severe. Dolly, for instance, had cancer of the colon and was admitted after becoming chronically incontinent at home. Her husband told me that, every time she had a severe bout of diarrhoea, she had begged him to help her take her own life. Dolly's requests for euthanasia continued during the first week of her stay in the hospice. Staff were unable to get her diarrhoea under control. In addition, she went into obstruction. The tumour mass expanded and blocked her colon and, as a consequence, digested food would reach her lower gut and then come back up as faecal vomit. Around the time Dolly went into total obstruction, staff observed a notable change in her behaviour. She stopped requesting euthanasia; in fact she stopped talking altogether. When members of the nursing staff came to turn her in bed or to attend to her care she would close her eyes and totally ignore them. As one nurse observed: 'it's as if she's shut the outside world out and herself off in the process'.

This type of 'switching off' has been identified elsewhere; for example, the response of victims in the Holocaust. Pines points to instances where women in this particular setting, 'overwhelmed by physical and emotional helplessness and despair, almost reached a state of psychic death' (1993: 185; see also Langer 1996), and uses Lifton's (1967) concept of 'psychic closing off' to indicate the loss of self that had occurred (1993: 180). Parallels can also be drawn with Martin's (1989) study of women suffering from brief periods of bodily trauma and unboundedness such as during menstruation, childbirth and caesarean section. These women, likewise, experienced altered and debased conceptions of self[3] (1989: 79–84; see also Grosz 1994), but because their bodily disruptions were only temporary – and thus reversible – they were able to regain a normal sense of self. Amongst many of the hospice patients with severely and irreversibly unbounded bodies I observed (and the Holocaust women discussed by Pines) the self appears to have more or less gone altogether, leaving little, if anything, but an empty body.

Other patients, like Annie, made more explicit attempts to 'switch themselves off' by requesting heavy sedation. Kath, for example, asked that she be moved to a side room and given a large dose of analgesics after commenting, on repeated occasions, that, 'you wouldn't put a dog through this'. Her message was clear and simple: it would be much more compassionate if the staff put her out of her misery. Some patients, like Deborah, refused to eat or drink, thereby accelerating their own demise; others, like Dolly, made direct requests for euthanasia. Stan, a patient with cancer of the prostate, began suffering from chronic diarrhoea about a week into his admission. He also had problems with his catheter which frequently became blocked because bits of tumour were being secreted in his urine. On a number of occasions he would wake up 'covered in my own dirt and wetness'. He repeatedly asked the staff to help him to die.

What all these examples highlight is that once a patient's body fell severely and irreversibly apart, she or he exhibited behaviour which suggests a loss of self. Such a phenomenon was perhaps most evident amongst those patients who 'switched off' and became disengaged from all events and relationships taking place around them (hence Deborah's daughter's comment that her mother had already 'gone' once she became withdrawn). Other patients sought external aid to achieve a complete withdrawal, such as requesting heavy sedation. Sedation, as we have seen in the previous chapter, renders a patient into a 'non-person' by removing his or capacity to 'act' and to interact with others; it constitutes what Fagerhaugh and Strauss have termed an imposed 'social death' (1977: 162). Some patients also made direct requests for euthanasia. Euthanasia, as Dworkin suggests, is the option of a person who chooses death after 'life in earnest … has ended' (1993: 3); it is a strategy for bringing forward physical death to concur more closely with the demise of the person/self (see Walter 1994; Seale 1998).

The material outlined here throws a number of complex issues into relief. Lee and Morgan argue that: 'To ask the question of what constitutes death is to ask also what separates life from death and at what point life may hold greater worth than death' (1994: xii). All the patients considered here exhibited behaviour (withdrawal from social and reciprocity networks) which suggests a loss of self, a form of 'social death' (see Chapter 5) which sometimes occurred several weeks prior to their physical cessation. These observations thus provide important insights into the relationship between body and self in contexts such as modern England. It would appear that the bounded body, as a literally physical condition, is both central and fundamental to selfhood, since we have seen something of the impossibility of retaining this status whilst having a body without boundaries (as we shall see below, the physically bounded body is important because of the ways in which personhood is constructed in modern 'Western' cultures). Thus, it could be argued that the hospice served on one level as 'fringe/liminal' space within which these 'non-persons', wavering 'between two worlds', remain buffered (Van Gennep 1972: 18).

The 'special status' accorded to patients with advanced cancer

Within medical and social science literatures, concern has been expressed about the fact that cancer patients are accorded a special status in relation to other persons (particularly older people) suffering from chronic degenerative diseases. Contemporary hospices are principally geared to care for patients with advanced cancer, whereas elderly and other patients with degenerative diseases – 'the disadvantaged dying' (Harris 1990) – are rarely included in planning services for continuing and terminal care (Clark 1993: 172; Cohen 1996). 'The disproportionate concentration of care on those dying of cancer', as Harris suggests, 'has created an underclass of dying people' (1990: 28). Seale (1989), likewise, observes that it is much easier to raise money for cancer services (e.g. for building a hospice) than for older people. However, no wholly satisfactory explanation has as yet been offered as to why this should be the case.

The special status accorded to cancer patients can perhaps be explained in part by the fact that the cancer death is commonly associated with the 'untimely' and hence 'tragic' death (Hockey 1990: 78).[4] In addition, what pits advanced cancer in contrast to other chronic degenerative conditions (e.g. arthritis or osteoporosis), and mental (e.g. Alzheimer's) and cardiac diseases is that life expectancy can be predicted with a fair degree of accuracy (Sudnow 1967: 67). Consequently, as Field notes, it is much easier to see patients with advanced malignant disease as 'dying' in both lay and medical perceptions (1996: 263).

Whilst observations such of these are clearly important, my findings suggest that an additional reason why institutionalised hospice care caters now more or less exclusively for cancer patients is because of the ways in which cancer, in its late stages, can severely affect the boundedness of a patient's body. Indeed, as we have seen above, there are strong grounds for arguing that inpatient hospices act as liminal spaces in which the unbounded body is both mediated and contained. It is significant, therefore, that amongst other categories of (non-cancer) patients, bodily unboundedness generally occurs less frequently and with less severity. Weisman, for example, has noted that a very different attitude pertains to the cardiac patient than to a patient with cancer. He explains this difference as stemming in part from the fact that cardio-vascular diseases are unlikely to affect a patient's body image, whereas cancer (and its treatment) often results in physical disfigurement (1979: 36–8). D. Morris similarly notes that chronic illness, accompanied by chronic pain, 'keep[s] a low profile by doggedly failing to convey the macabre glory of deformity ... [it] attacks millions of people without *leaving outward signs of damage*' (1991: 66, emphasis added).

The sequestration of the unbounded body: an ethnographic and theoretical discussion

One obvious question clearly remains to be addressed: why the sequestration of the unbounded body is deemed both appropriate and necessary within contexts such as contemporary England. It is thus to this issue that I now turn.

When carers discussed their reasons for wanting a patient to come into the hospice, their comments revealed one particularly notable theme. Carers, as a general rule, did not seem to be explicitly concerned about the fact that a patient was dying: on the contrary, the main reason they gave for wanting a patient to be admitted was because they felt repelled by the patient being incontinent, vomiting, and/or emitting other bodily fluids within their own homes.[5] As the wife of one patient put it:

He started having a lot of problems with vomiting. You just never knew when it was going to happen. All of a sudden it would just come pouring out. It went everywhere ... all over his bed, all over the carpet. It was disgusting.

Another wife offered the following comment:

> Things got very difficult after he became incontinent. I had
> to help him change his pads. It made me feel really sick. ...
> Sometimes he had an accident and it went all over the
> place. I still can't get the stench of urine out of the carpet.
> ... I'm so glad he's in here now.

Carers' perceptions were also often shared by patients themselves.
As Annie's case has already highlighted, patients often felt that
home did not afford an appropriate space for their bodily
disintegration, since the experience of being incontinent in front of
family and friends could be extremely distressing and humiliating
to them.[6]

The breakdown of the body's boundedness, furthermore, was
often accompanied by the emission of smells. Smell was a perpetual
problem within the hospice: on a number of occasions, staff kept
aromatherapy oil burners running throughout the day and night in
an attempt to veil the odour of excreta, vomit and rotting flesh. It
quickly came to my attention that the odours released from
patients' disintegrating bodies not only precipitated their admission
to the hospice, but, in addition, often brought about a further
marginalisation within the building itself. I observed that smell
created a boundary around a patient, repelling others away. On
several occasions, patients were driven out of the wards after
another patient had been heavily incontinent in bed. For example,
Bill became doubly incontinent shortly before he died. Another
patient in his ward, Brian, took himself off to the day room early
on in the morning and staunchly refused to re-enter the ward until
the evening. I initially assumed that Brian wished to avoid Bill
because he did not want to be in the same space as a dying patient.
However, this misapprehension was quickly dispelled. Brian
explained that he did not have any difficulties being exposed to
people who were dying: he had fought in World War II and,
consequently, had witnessed many deaths first hand. Instead, Brian
pointed to the 'terrible smell': 'I've worked on a pig farm and not
smelt anything as bad as this.' A similar view was expressed by
Doris, who, as described above, pressed for her own discharge after
Annie deteriorated significantly in the bed next to her.

Sometimes, staff attempted to manage problems of smell by
transferring a patient to a side room, thereby enabling the odours
emitted from his or her body to be contained within a more
bounded space – Annie being a good case in point. To take another
example, a male patient, Ron, was moved after it was reported that

'he smelt like dog shit'. One of the nurses added that, 'you couldn't go into his ward this morning without squirting lemon aerosol in front of your nose'. Other patients were admitted directly to side rooms because of anticipated problems with odour. Sydney, for instance, was placed in a single room because he had a fungating tumour. The smell in fact proved to be so repellent that his wife refused to go into his room from the time of his admission until his death six days later.

Douglas, in her analysis of pollution concepts and taboos, argues for a symbolic classificatory approach to culturally embedded ideas of defilement and disorder. Concepts of 'dirt', she suggests, emerge in situations where a set of ordered relations and classificatory schema are directly contravened. Hence, pollution behaviour 'is the reaction which condemns any object or idea likely to confuse or contradict cherished classifications' (1984: 36). Douglas' approach can thus be usefully applied to provide some insights into why intolerance of bodily emissions and smells has become such a marked feature of the contemporary 'deodorised' 'West'. Whilst the carers observed in my study expressed revulsion towards the odours and substances emitted from the bodies of 'unbounded' patients, both Classen *et al.* (1994) and Corbin (1986) provide rich accounts which suggest that historically (especially in the medieval period) mainstream European social life was pervaded by the smells of bodies, bodily emissions and other pungent odours; a phenomenon which has been described with particular vividness in Süskind's (1987) novel *Perfume*. As Classen *et al.* observe, 'odours cannot easily be contained, they escape and cross boundaries, blending different olfactory wholes' (1994: 4). Being inherently transgressive of boundaries, smells are thus opposed to 'our modern linear world view, with its emphasis on privacy, discrete divisions and superficial interactions' (1994: 5). Such a perspective, then, may help to explain why patients with un-bounded bodies were sequestered within the hospice. Hospices, it could be argued, serve to impose order upon disorder through enclosing and containing the odours emitted from patients' disintegrating bodies within a bounded space. It requires little further imagination to suggest that the walls of the hospice served as the boundaries of a patient's body in situations where a patient lacked the corporeal capacity for 'self-containment'.

Yet it would be unwise to accord too much credence to the suggestion made by Classen *et al.* (1994) and Corbin (1986) that the modern 'West' has become intolerant of odours *per se*. One needs only to look at the widespread use of products designed to make people 'smell good' (for example, perfumes, after-shaves and scented soaps) to recognise that it is not smell as such that is denigrated in contemporary 'Western' contexts: it is certain *specific* types of smell. Indeed, as I will now go on to examine, the negative reaction provoked by the bodily odours and substances emitted from patients' bodies could actually be understood as stemming primarily from the way in which the person/self is constructed and conceived in modern 'Western' contexts. By highlighting the centrality of the physically bounded body to such a conception, furthermore, we shall see an example in which the 'Western' person/self appears to conform to 'rhetorics of individuality'.

As I have already indicated in the previous chapter, it is a now a well-rehearsed argument within the anthropological and sociological literature that the body, and experiential modes of embodiment, are culturally elaborated and culturally embedded products. Following on from Mauss' observations on 'techniques of the body' (1992) [1934], Douglas, for example, has argued for a dialectical relationship between the body and society within any given cultural milieu. Whilst the body can act as a 'model for society' by affording 'a source of symbols for other complex structures' (1984: 115), Douglas also suggests that the 'social body constrains the way the physical body is perceived' (1970: 65). Hence, it is through the body, and the ways in which the body is deployed and modified that socially appropriate self-understandings are created and reproduced. Douglas, needless to say, could be criticised for making somewhat generalising claims about the character of human bodies and boundaries: for example, her suggestion that the 'body is a model which can stand for any bounded system. Its boundaries can represent any boundaries which are threatened or precarious' (1984: 115). As Taylor's (n.d.) and Meigs' (1984) ethnographic observations (discussed later) usefully highlight, bodies are not in fact universally conceived as physically bounded entities. There are, nonetheless, grounds for suggesting that Douglas' analysis remains both relevant and helpful to studies of 'Western' embodiment because it would appear that her notion of body boundaries is (ethnocentrically) linked to contemporary 'Western' conceptions of personhood.

A similar argument to Douglas' is presented by Bourdieu, who points to the inter-relationship between embodied activities and the 'habitus' within which they are located. The body, he suggests, enters into the production of the habitus; it acts as the mediator between social structures and individual action, being shaped by the former and itself regulating the latter (1978: 834). As I noted in Chapter 3, Foucault also treats the body as an emergent product of cultural norms and regulations, although he is primarily concerned with the body as a site of political 'subjection' inscribed by systems of power. For Foucault, power relations impinge directly upon bodies so as to construct them as 'docile' and 'useful'. Yet the power exercised over, and through, the body does not necessarily have to be the privilege of a dominant class. As Foucault goes on to suggest, through the normalising practices that accompany the standardisation of the industrial process, power becomes diffused everywhere, amongst the dominated as well as the dominant (1991: 184).

The work of the above academics can thus be fed into, and used to support, Elias' argument that contemporary 'Western' constructions of the body as a peculiarly intimate and private thing are neither natural nor innate, but the product of a long, gradual and historically specific 'civilising process' (1994). This process, which extended over many centuries, involved the gradual elaboration and internalisation, in the form of self controls, of a whole series of taboos and precepts regulating such things as bodily functions and bodily exposure. As a consequence, a number of 'natural functions' such as defecating, urinating and spitting which had previously been public acts were eliminated from social life and displaced 'behind the scenes' (1994: 114). As Elias further suggests, the privatisation of bodily functions did not occur uniformly across society: bodily taboos and affect controls first became commonplace amongst the upper classes in Western Europe, and slowly filtered down to, and became established amongst, the bourgeoisie, followed later by the lower social classes.

Elias thus traces a gradual historical transition from an 'open', 'incomplete' body, to a body with clearly defined boundaries, isolated, alone, and fenced off from other bodies (Elias 1994: 56; Fontaine 1978: 245); a phenomenon also pointed to by Bakhtin (1968) in the distinction he draws between the 'grotesque' and the 'classical' body. What is particularly pertinent in Elias' historical account is the relationship that can be drawn between the emergence of the bounded body as central to contemporary 'Western' conceptions of the person and the rise of individualism. Crawford, for example, stresses the relationship between the ascetic individualism of the Protestant Reformation and the construction of the body as 'healthy', 'enclosed' and 'disciplined'. He suggests that the 'Protestant temperament' of austerity, coupled with a 'work ethic' has inculcated a predisposition towards applied entrepreneurial activity and disciplined saving. Such a phenomenon, as he further points out, has also led to an emphasis upon personal discipline, autonomy and self-responsibility (1994: 1349; see also Foucault 1991: 138). Crawford's argument thus closely parallels Douglas' assertion that the body can act as a 'text' which reflects and reproduces the concerns, values and preoccupations of the particular culture within which it is located (see above).[7] Self-control, in effect, has become mapped onto, and experienced within, the physical body as *self-containment*. Hence, Bordo's observation that the contemporary 'Western' body ideal – achieved through activities such as dieting and 'working out' – has become one which is 'absolutely tight, contained, "bolted down" ' (1993: 190). The 'quest for firm bodily margins' (1993: 191), she suggests, can be understood within a cultural context in which 'the firm, developed body has become a symbol of the correct *attitude*; it means that one "cares" about oneself and how one appears to others, suggesting will power, energy, control over infantile impulse, the ability to "shape your life" ' (1993: 195, original emphasis). In a similar vein, Gell develops Anzieu's idea of 'character armour' to explain the contemporary 'Western' preoccupation with body-building. Body-building, according to Gell's reading of Anzieu's work, serves as a means of constructing 'an extra-resilient second skin around the "real self" ' (1993: 34), and thus fulfils the requirements of the 'individual' who needs to be 'protected' and 'sealed off' (1993: 38). Benson, likewise, argues that current cultural preoccupations with practices such as body-building and tattooing embody 'a fear of fragmentation, a fear of sociality and connection and a celebration and obsessional enactment of ideas of autonomous will and self, centring on the idea of fortifying and sealing the body' (Benson n.d.).

Careful scrutiny of the ethnographic literature provides a further indication of the culturally as well as historically specific nature of the bounded, sealed body of the contemporary 'Western' person. Cross-cultural comparison suggests that, in societies where relationships are not governed by capitalist and industrial modes of production, persons, bodies and bodily processes may be constructed, conceived and evaluated in different ways. The work of Strathern, in particular, draws our attention to the notion that, in Melanesian societies, the person is not viewed as a discrete monad, ontologically separate from others, but, rather, as a relational entity, which is never completely whole, and neither singular nor plural (Strathern 1988). Within such societies, identities are fluid and fragmentary, since it is through a constant flux of gift exchanges that a person habitually adds to and produces other persons. In effect, persons relate to one another through various aspects of themselves and not as integrated and bounded units.

Both Taylor (n.d.) and Meigs (1984) have produced ethnographic studies which suggest that, in cultural settings where personhood is conceived of as permeable and plural, bodies are, likewise, constructed and experienced as porous and uncontained. For example, Meigs describes how amongst the Hau of the Highlands of Papua New Guinea, identity is generated and defined more in terms of fluids and scents than in terms of external anatomy. Hau conceive of emissions from the body (such as sweat, vomit, excreta) as infused with a person's self and as carriers of the owner's essence (1984: 111). Consequently, persons may relate to one another through their body fluids: a man, for example, smears his sweat, oil and vomit over the bodies of his real and classificatory kin, since such substances are believed to be ingested through the pores of their skin and to cause growth (1984: 109). The 'Rwandans' studied by Taylor, likewise, conceive of bodily emissions as extensions of the person. Taylor, for example, describes a ritual in which a new born child is presented to members of the family and local community for the first time. During the ritual, all the children present are asked to bestow a name upon the new-born. The children are then given a meal termed 'to eat the baby's excrement', since the food they consume is mixed with a small amount of the baby's faecal matter. For Taylor's 'Rwandans', this ritual celebrates the fact that the baby's body has been found to be an open conduit, an adequate vessel for perpetuating the process of 'flow'. As Taylor suggests, 'in a sense, the baby's faeces are its first gift and the members of his [sic] age class are its first recipients. The children at this ceremony incorporate the child into their group by ingesting one of his bodily products' (n.d.).

It would, needless to say, be problematic to posit a simple dichotomy between a bounded 'Western' person and a 'dividual', fluid non-Western one. However, there would seem to be grounds for suggesting that in cultural contexts where persons are not necessarily conceived as 'individuals', substances emitted from the body, whether they are attributed a positive or negative value, are not understood as 'waste' or 'dirt' in the same way as in contemporary 'Western' contexts (Meigs 1984: 112; Douglas 1984: 121). Indeed, as Corbin argues, the contemporary 'Western' perception of body odours and body substances as 'filth'[8] (that is, as something to be avoided and disposed of) should be understood as stemming from a new 'spatiality of the body', which has developed in parallel with the emergence of the concept of the 'individual' (1986: 61). It is highly significant, as Corbin further notes, that 'hygiene reforms' geared to 'privatising human waste' and 'deodorising' public and private spaces predated Pasteur's germ theory of disease, but occurred concurrently with the early stages of the historical development of individualism.[9] Much the same observation is made by Elias who suggests that the closure of the body, achieved through the isolation of natural functions from public life, was originally grounded in 'moral' concerns, and only later came to be understood as necessary for 'hygienic' reasons (1994: 123). In other words, advances in science and medicine cannot be accorded a deterministic role in the development of modern 'hygiene sensibilities'; instead we should understand these sensibilities as being more symbolic in nature, stemming, in the first instance, from the construction of the body as a self-contained, physically bounded entity.[10]

It is now possible to understand further why patients with unbounded bodies were sequestered within the hospice. As the above analysis suggests, within modern 'Western' contexts, the unbounded body is perceived symbolically both as a locus and a source of 'dirt'; as 'matter out of place' (Douglas 1984: 35). (Hence the repulsion carers often expressed towards caring for 'unbounded' patients, and managing their body secretions and emissions, within their own homes.) It certainly seems to be no coincidence that patients, carers and staff members alike often employed animal metaphors to describe and account for the experiences of patients with unbounded bodies. Recall the following quotes: 'you wouldn't put a dog through this'; 'he smelt like dog shit'; 'I've worked on a pig farm and not smelt anything as bad as this.' The association between 'unbounded' patients and 'fetid' animals festering in their own dung was very evident in my fieldwork observations. If we return to Douglas' argument that 'dirt' offends against 'order', it is evident that contemporary hospices serve to remove patient's dirt, and the patient *as dirt*, from the mainstream of society.[11]

The unbounded body and the loss of the person

The above discussions lend further insights as to why patients with severely unbounded bodies evinced, and experienced, a loss of self. As this material has highlighted, the bounded, physically sealed body has become central to concepts of person/self within 'Western' contexts such as England. Hence, it could be argued that patients with unbounded bodies lost one of the criteria for personhood by virtue of their lacking the corporeal capacity for 'self-containment'. It has, indeed, been recognised within the social scientific literature that bodily closure, achieved through continence, is a necessary means by which entry into 'full person' status is now gained and sustained. Hockey and James, for instance, have noted that one of the central markers of a child's progress from infancy to maturity is the ability to control bowel and bladder functions (1993: 85). In a similar vein, Mitteness and Barker have observed that incontinence amongst elderly people is frequently thought to symbolise, 'that the elder is no longer an adult person but is on the road to the ultimate in disorderliness and decrepitude, to becoming a nonperson' (1995: 206). They further observe that, 'there is a general tendency amongst physicians to assume that once incontinence becomes flagrant, that is, public and therefore no longer able to be ignored, institutionalization [i.e. sequestration] is the best – or only – treatment option available' (1995: 204).

It is perhaps significant to note that young infants, who also have unbounded bodies, are also subjected to sequestering practices to some extent. For example, there are many public places from which infants are excluded and other spaces (such as nurseries) designed specifically for them. As a consequence, the adults most likely to have intimate contact with an 'unbounded' infant and his or her body substances are the infant's parents. It could be argued that, because babies and young children are not fully grown, they are thought, to some extent, to be an extension of their parents' bodies; an integral part of their own selfhood. Thus, parents do not express the same abhorrence towards a baby's body substances as they would towards those from an 'unbounded' adult, because a baby's body products and emissions 'merge' with their own to some extent.

Gender issues are also raised in the threat of bodily unboundedness to personhood. Women's bodies remain unbounded throughout much of their younger adult lives as a result of menstruation which, unlike defecation and urination, cannot be controlled but merely blocked. Grosz has argued that in the modern 'West', women's bodies and sexualities have become structured and lived in terms which not only differentiate them from men's, but which also, to some extent, position them in a relation of passive dependence and secondariness to men (1994: 202). This phenomenon, she suggests, stems from the construction and inscription of women's corporeality 'not only as a lack or absence', but, with more complexity, as 'a mode of seepage' (1994: 203). Hence there exists 'a broadly common coding of the female body as a body which leaks, which bleeds, which is at the mercy of hormonal and reproductive functions' (1994: 204).

The hospice: a 'no place'

As I examined in Chapter 1, a substantial literature argues that death and dying are one of our main cultural taboos within contemporary 'Western' contexts (see, for example, Ariès 1974, 1981; Gorer 1965; Moller 1996). Within this framework the contemporary hospice movement, despite its own overt goal of humanising the dying process, is frequently understood as a further exemplar of the widespread social desire to sequester and hide the processes of death and dying from the mainstream of social life (see, for instance, Mellor 1993). The above observations and analyses, however, suggest that this interpretation is far from adequate since, as we have seen, hospices do not veil the dying process *per se*. On the contrary, there is an increasing trend towards hospices sequestering very specific types of dying and very specific kinds of patients: those who have bodies which are unbounded.

The above observations could thus be used to argue that contemporary hospices in fact employ one set of taboos, that is, their stereotype as 'houses of death' (Kastenbaum and Aisenberg 1974) or 'little pockets in which our culture hides the terminally ill and muffles the voice of death' (Scott 1994: 37), to veil a second more important set of taboos: those associated with the ways in which a number of patients admitted to hospices actually deteriorate, rot away and die. Issues of dirt, decay, disintegration and smell are rarely, if ever, written about by hospice professionals or covered in media representations of hospice care. On the contrary, such phenomena are usually 'glossed over' as 'symptoms' requiring 'control'. Hospices practise a type of care now termed 'palliative'. Palliative care is formally defined as:

active total care offered to a patient with a progressive disease and their family when it is recognised that the illness is no longer curable, in order to concentrate on the quality of life and the alleviation of distressing symptoms within the framework of a co-ordinated service.

(Standing Medical Advisory Committee and Standing Nursing and Midwifery Advisory Committee 1993)

As Scott points out, however, the actual word 'palliative' is derived from the Latin noun pallium, meaning 'cloak'. Palliate means, quite literally, 'to cover with or as with a cloak ... to hide, conceal, disguise' (1994: 37). The fieldwork observations described in this chapter suggest that the latter understanding and use of the term is most salient in understanding the contemporary role of hospices.

In this respect, the hospice involved in my study could be understood not simply as a liminal space but rather as a 'no place', in the sense used by Vialles in her discussion of the development of the modern abattoir in France. For Vialles the construction of the abattoir as a 'no-place' resulted from 'the profound shift in sensibilities with regard to such realities as death (human and animal), suffering, violence, waste and disease' (1994: 19) These 'realities' became something that the 'general public neither needs *nor wishes to know*' (1994: 22, emphasis added). Hence the slaughtering of animals became a process confined within the abattoir; something that 'must be invisible (ideally: non existent). It must be as if it were not' (1994: 22). Understanding the hospice as a 'no place', that is, as a space within which the taboo processes of bodily disintegration and decay are sequestered, allows it to be understood as a central part of contemporary English culture. Setting these phenomena apart from mainstream society, it could be argued, enables certain ideas about living, personhood and the hygienic, sanitised, bounded body (Meyer 1991: 265) to be symbolically enforced and maintained. It may, indeed, be no coincidence that the hospice where I conducted fieldwork was located on the site of the city's former 'isolation' or fever hospital.

It is not surprising, therefore, that the 'dirty processes' palliated within the bounded setting of the hospice, proved to be very disturbing and upsetting to those people who *actually* witnessed patients' deterioration and eventual deaths firsthand. It was not uncommon for family and friends to suggest that they were more distressed by the ways in which a patient died than the fact of death itself. For example, Deborah's daughter (Deborah was one of the two patients discussed above who had a fistula) suggested that she had not been excessively upset by the fact of her mother's death: 'After all, my mother [aged 79] had already had a good, long life. She actually said herself that if cancer hadn't taken her something else would have instead.' She was, however, having great difficulties coming to terms with the 'difficult and dirty exit my mother endured'; she did not think her mother had 'any dignity at the end'. A similar view was expressed by the husband of another patient in the hospice, Claire, who had advanced breast cancer and gross lymphoedema in her arms and legs. He frequently pointed to the 'brutal' way in which Claire's cancer was eating her body away. In one particularly emotional outpouring he told me that he had been in the armed forces for seventeen and a half years and had witnessed many deaths. Yet he had never seen anything quite so 'cruel and disgusting' as what was happening to his wife. The husband of another patient suggested that it would have been much easier if his wife had been 'run over by a bus' than to see her 'rot away so slowly'.

Concluding remarks

The above discussions thus throw new light upon the function of the contemporary inpatient hospices, together with providing deeper insights into why hospice/palliative care is largely confined to patients with advanced cancer and who experience 'difficult' symptoms. It also points to an inadequacy in much of the academic literature on death and dying. This literature tends to build its theoretical paradigms upon assumptions of homogeneous categories such as 'the dying patient' and 'the dying process' (see Elias 1985; Hockey 1990; Ariès 1981; Moller 1996). To explain the marginalisation of patients within hospices and other institutions simply because they are 'dying' would seem to be somewhat unsatisfactory. Rather, this chapter has pointed to the importance of considering the body and the disease processes taking place within it and upon its surfaces as a central and reflexive part of analysis.

With such observations in mind, I will conclude by briefly exploring and critiquing the analytical frameworks and findings of recent research which has examined the impact of patient deaths upon fellow hospice patients. As I have already indicated in earlier chapters, a number of professionals involved with the modern hospice movement had, by the time of my research, begun to question the practice of keeping dying patients in communal wards. This line of questioning prompted studies to be conducted by Honeybun *et al.* (1992) and Payne *et al.* (1996), who explored the impact of death on fellow patients by comparing psychological morbidity and perceptions of comfort and/or distress between hospice patients who had witnessed a death during their stay and those who had not. (Patients were assessed using the Hospital Anxiety and Depression scale, an Events Checklist and a semi-structured interview.) Both studies found that patients who had witnessed a death were 'significantly less depressed' than those who had not. It was also observed that patients rated the death of another patient as a more comforting than distressing experience.

Not surprisingly, the authors of these particular studies concluded that patients did benefit from witnessing the death of a fellow patient, and hence that, 'all other things being equal, retaining the dying patient in the room with other patients would appear to be in the interests of these other patients' (Honeybun *et al.* 1992: 72). One can thus see the results of these particular studies as a powerful endorsement of the hospice movement's practice of an open confrontation with death; a practice which is achieved in part by continuing to design hospices to house the majority of patients in wards rather than in side rooms.

Whilst I certainly do not wish to dismiss the findings of these studies in their entirety, the authors' underlying presuppositions are in need of careful and critical scrutiny. One of the most problematic aspects of their research stems from the way 'dying' is both assumed to be, and treated as, a homogenous process. It may well be the case that patients do benefit from witnessing some types of deaths; for example, those in which patients 'drift off peacefully' (see Chapter 4), yet, as the ethnographic material in this book has vividly highlighted, not all patients die in such seemingly dignified ways. As we have seen, in cases where patients' bodies become severely unbounded prior to death, and those in which they become very paranoid or confused, other patients may actively go out of their way to avoid being in the same space as them (and indeed staff will often attempt to hide 'bad deaths' away in side rooms). Clearly then there are certain types of dying which patients do not actually wish to observe, or benefit from observing; types of dying, needless to say, that are glossed over in research that makes generalising claims, based upon generalised categories and assumptions.[12] The findings of both studies in fact have little, if anything, helpful to say to staff with regard to the very real dilemmas they confront in caring for patients who experience complex and distressing symptoms in the final stages approaching death.

Such dilemmas, needless to say, are likely to be heightened in the future, if the observations and trends highlighted in this chapter are anything to go by. With the progressive shift that is occurring towards the care of dying patients in 'the community', inpatient hospices are progressively becoming enclaves for those types of dying which people cannot – and do not – want to witness directly. Hospices, in other words, are now catering for very different patients to those who formed the focus of concern when the movement was first founded in the 1960s. In light of such changes, one cannot help but question whether it is going to continue to remain helpful and viable to advocate an open confrontation with death within hospices if this means, in practice, that patients, increasingly, are going to be exposed to deaths which they find extremely upsetting. It may well prove to be the case that patients, in the future, would actually benefit more from being cared for in hospices which are designed to accommodate a higher proportion within single rooms.

5

INVISIBLE SUFFERING
The social death

Introduction

In this chapter, the body is allowed to recede temporarily into the background to enable a second, related way in which patients experienced a loss of self to be explored: a loss of self which stemmed from a loss of relationships. Such a theme was first highlighted in Chapter 2, in which the experiences of patients admitted to the day care service were examined. A number of day care patients had become very isolated and demoralised because family and friends had started withdrawing from them. Such withdrawal stemmed partly from the stigmatising effects of illness, coupled with the knowledge of family and friends that the patient was going to die. Yet, as Chapter 2 also described, patients' experiences of social isolation could also be understood as resulting from the ways in which their social and temporal perceptions had ceased to be enmeshed with those of the people around them. Patients, in a sense, had become drawn into ways of seeing and experiencing the world with which family and friends could not empathise. Both parties, as a consequence, felt increasingly alienated and estranged from one another; the common ground between them had begun to dissipate and ebb away.

Day care patients were generally at an earlier stage in their illness and deterioration than those admitted to the hospice and, as this chapter highlights, the problem of becoming alienated and dislodged from networks of interpersonal relationships was experienced in particularly marked and distressing ways amongst the latter. A number of hospice patients indicated that they wished they had died earlier; a situation which suggested that they had experienced a form of social death prior to their physical demise (see, for example, Seale 1998). Yet, whilst it was common for patients to encounter the problem of 'living too long', there was also a small subgroup within the hospice who 'died too soon'. In these rare instances, patients remained socially intact, that is, fully embedded within networks of relationships until the point at which they died. As I highlight later, the deaths of these particular patients were considered to be especially upsetting and 'tragic' by staff and family alike. The distressing nature of such deaths stemmed from the fact that both the patient, and his or her family, had had insufficient time to make the necessary social and emotional adjustments prior to the death.

The body is intentionally allowed to elide from view in the first sections of this chapter as a strategy for making visible the erosive effects that a loss of relationships had upon a patient's self. Such a strategy, though analytically useful, presents a partial picture. As the chapter goes on to examine, patients' bodily deterioration could also often be implicated – either directly or indirectly – in the processes which led to their removal from relationships and thus to their social deaths. A central observation thus developed is that bodies cannot necessarily be isolated from relationships and, likewise, relationships cannot, in practice, be considered in isolation from bodies.

The chapter concludes with an analysis which provides insights into why patients appeared to become 'disinvested' of their gender at a fairly early stage in their deterioration, whereas, in contrast, they generally seemed to retain their class attributes and tastes more or less right up until the point at which they actually died.

'Living too long'

Whilst explicit requests for euthanasia were comparatively rare within the hospice, it was not uncommon for patients to indicate that they wished that they had died sooner and, in some cases, to employ strategies such as refusing food and drink to accelerate the arrival of death. Medical staff tried, whenever possible, to be sensitive to the needs and wishes of patients: if, for example, a patient had developed a chest infection and that patient had already indicated that she or he was 'wanting' or 'ready to go', staff would generally not treat it with antibiotics. As I indicated in Chapter 3, sedation was also used as a means of reducing or eliminating patients' distress by erasing their awareness of self and environment. Whilst strategies such as those just described were commonly employed in cases where patients suffered from the humiliating effects of bodily unboundedness, I also observed another distinct subgroup who seemed 'ready to die' but for whom distressing physical symptoms were not necessarily the primary factors which caused their distress. Such patients, as I now go on to examine, suffered from social isolation in an extreme form: they were described somewhat poignantly by the hospice's occupational therapist as being those who had 'no one to love them or care about them'.

Case study – Rose

Rose, a woman aged 71, was first diagnosed with non-Hodgkin's lymphoma in 1991 and was given a prognosis of between one and two years by her hospital consultant. At the time, she was living in Scotland where she had moved with her husband in 1970, after he had been transferred there by his employer. In 1980, her husband died suddenly in a car accident, a death with which Rose felt that she had never fully come to terms. After she became ill, with nothing to keep her in Scotland, she decided to move back to England so that she could be closer to her son and daughter and her grandchildren. She moved into a rented bungalow close to her daughter's house.

Rose first became known to me through day care (May 1994), by which time she had already lived considerably longer than her hospital consultant had predicted. Her sense of isolation at home was very apparent: she had not made any friends since she returned from Scotland, and the only person who visited her on a regular basis was her daughter who helped her with her cooking, cleaning and laundry. Her son and daughter-in-law had originally come to see her on a weekly basis (they lived about ten miles from Rose's bungalow), but their visits attenuated away after about a year.

The strain of looking after Rose on a long-term basis had clearly had a substantial impact upon her daughter who, by then, had been her main carer for more than three years. She broke down in tears in an interview I held with her, pointing, in particular, to the tensions that had begun to develop in her own marriage. Whilst her husband had initially been very understanding and supportive, he had come to resent the fact that she had no time to spend with him and their three young children. The daughter suggested that they both felt 'cheated' because Rose had lived 'for much longer than we'd ever expected'. She also spoke of the resentment she felt towards her brother for 'walking away and getting on with his own life' as soon as 'the novelty of mum being sick faded off'.

Rose was finally admitted to the hospice in April 1995 after she developed pneumonia. Her illness left her extremely weak and lethargic; she was so weak in fact that she and her family were warned by medical staff that she might not live for more than a few weeks. Rose, at this stage, expressed the wish to be discharged home for a short time, suggesting that she would like to say her 'good-byes' properly to her family before returning to the hospice to die. As she was not well enough to return to her bungalow, her daughter and son-in-law agreed that she could move temporarily into their own home. Hospice staff arranged for a home care nurse to visit twice a day to assist with her care.

Rose returned to the hospice after a ten-day stay at home. She told me that her visit had been 'an enormous success'; everyone had been extremely kind to her and she had been treated 'like a queen'. In a meeting with the hospice social worker, however, her daughter made it clear that her mother's visit had been far from successful from her own point of view. Rose, apparently, had embraced a 'death bed role' in its entirety, and had summoned all her immediate and distant relatives to her bed-side, telling them that she had very little time left and wanted to say her farewells. Whilst Rose had been lavished with attention as a consequence, her daughter had found the whole situation extremely stressful and upsetting. She complained that the telephone and the door bell had not stopped ringing throughout the ten-day period of her mother's stay.

After Rose returned to the hospice, she did not deteriorate in the way the doctors had predicted. In fact, much to everyone's surprise, her condition began to improve. This left the hospice staff in a somewhat difficult and embarrassing situation: as one of the doctors pointed out at the time, they no longer had a 'dying woman' on their hands. He went on to speculate that Rose could, quite possibly, now live for several more months. Rose was discharged a couple of days later because the bed she was occupying needed to be freed for emergency admissions. She returned to her daughter's home.

Rose's stay at home lasted only for a matter of days before she was unexpectedly readmitted to the hospice. On her arrival, she was extremely subdued: she told me that things at home 'had not been the same as last time', but was very reluctant to offer any further explanation. I only found out what had actually happened when her case was discussed in a multi-disciplinary team meeting held the following week. Two days after her discharge, the hospice social worker and one of the doctors had visited Rose and her daughter and son-in-law at home to discuss her future care arrangements. During this visit, they explained that they would not be able to provide Rose with long-term care within the hospice because it was only a short-stay facility: suitable arrangements would therefore have to be made so that she could be cared for at home.

At this stage in the discussions, Rose's daughter burst into tears. She complained that she had reached a state of total exhaustion, and also spoke openly of her resentment that she had spent so much time caring for her mother that she had not been able to watch her own children grow up. Both she and her husband made it clear that they were neither willing, nor able, to look after Rose any longer. Rose, who was present in the room at the time, immediately broke down herself, and insisted on returning to the hospice straight away. In the circumstances, staff had no choice but to readmit her.

On her readmission, Rose refused to talk to any of the nurses. During the first few days, she also declined all food and nursing care (e.g. a bed bath). Whenever a member of staff entered the ward, she closed her eyes and pretended to be asleep. On the rare occasions that I coaxed her into talking, she spoke of her sadness, suggesting that she might as well 'give up'.

No-one came to see her apart from her daughter, who occasionally made a brief visit during the afternoon. Rose was normally asleep at this time of day, and the daughter often chose to leave immediately rather than waiting until her mother woke up. During one such visit she told me that she was not in the least bit surprised that Rose had no other visitors. As far as the rest of her family were concerned, they had said their final 'good-byes' to her the first time she was discharged from the hospice. The daughter also complained that Rose had become 'a very manipulative person; as hard as nails under the surface'. Her mother, she said, had been claiming that she was dying for more than four years and, consequently, the whole family had finally run out of sympathy for her. The hospice's nursing staff, however, expressed a more compassionate view: the problem, as they saw it, was quite simply that Rose had 'lived for too long'.

Rose was not discharged from the hospice because, initially, there was nowhere to send her. Staff did set plans in motion to move her into residential care, but she died shortly before they were finalised. About a week before she died, Rose started talking about euthanasia and offered one of nursing assistants twenty pounds 'to get me out of here'. Her last words were shared with a cleaner a few hours before she slipped into a coma. She had a couple of cuddly toys in her locker and suggested that the cleaner should take them home and give them to her own grand-children. Rose died in a ward without any family and friends present.

In the above case study it appears that Rose's distress stemmed from the fact that she had 'lived too long' which, in practice, meant that she had become fully dislodged from her network of kinship and other interpersonal relationships. This process began with the death of her husband some fifteen years previously, and eventually culminated in the total withdrawal of all her family several weeks before she finally died. Her family's withdrawal resulted in large part from the fact that they had prepared themselves psychologically and emotionally for a death which they believed would occur a considerable time before it did. Indeed, whilst Rose was given a prognosis of between one and two years in 1991, she did not actually die until 1995. Her family also experienced a further 'false start' after she developed pneumonia and then made an unexpected recovery. By that stage, the strain experienced by Rose's main carer, her daughter, had become overwhelming. In order to preserve her relationships with her children, and to salvage a marriage which was rapidly falling apart, she was left with little choice but to abandon her role as carer and to break ties with the mother whom she felt she had failed.

Rose's sense of sadness and abandonment was further heightened because hospice staff were unable to promise her a 'temporary surrogate family' and 'safe haven' until she died. The possibility of a discharge into a residential home loomed large right up until the point at which she finally slipped into a coma. Rose's refusal to talk to the nurses and other staff could thus be understood as her response to what she saw as yet another painful rejection.

It would appear, then, that during the final weeks of her life Rose had entered a state of social death, wherein her family and others had started treating her as if she were 'as good as dead' (see Glaser and Strauss 1966; Sudnow 1967). Rose herself expressed a clear lack of interest in continuing to live after it became apparent to her that she had ceased to have an active influence in the lives of the people she had known and cared about.

Such a problem of social death was encountered by a number of hospice patients, though it was especially common amongst older patients and can be understood as stemming in part from their position in the life course (see, for example, Hazan 1980; Kearl 1989: 464). A number of older patients admitted to the hospice were described by staff as having 'already turned their faces to the wall and given up' which, in practice, meant that they showed no desire to continue living. Such patients had typically outlived their peer and sibling groups, and many also had no involvement with children (if they had them) or other surviving family members and friends. Elsie, for example, was an 80-year-old spinster with no living relatives, who was admitted for a week's respite after her warden accommodation had burnt down. She had been diagnosed with breast cancer three years previously and, at the time, had staunchly refused all treatment despite the fact that she had been told that she had a realistic chance of making a full recovery. Whilst she was in the hospice her sense of unhappiness and despondency became very apparent: she repeatedly told the nurses that she wanted to die. As she put it movingly: 'I always thought I was going to die when I was seventy-five. I'm old and *I'm alone.* What's the purpose in that?' (emphasis added). Arthur, similarly, was 70 and lived alone. He had only one surviving relative: a niece who had emigrated to New Zealand some years previously. His admission to the hospice took place after his district nurse became aware that he had stopped eating and answering his telephone. Apparently, he had passed his days sitting in a chair in his living room, staring at the walls. During his ten-day stay in the hospice, staff were unable to 'revitalise his interest in living'. Whilst the occupational therapist tried to encourage him to become more active, suggesting that he should read some books and listen to tapes, Arthur held a very different opinion. He complained that, whenever she visited him, he had to grit his teeth to prevent himself from cursing her out loud: all he wanted to do was to sit quietly beside his bed. Arthur told me that he objected to other people's interference, and, if he had been given a choice, he would have preferred to have been left alone at home to die.

Some hospice patients encountered the problem of 'living too long', even when they did have relatives and friends who were alive and living locally. As Rose's case study highlighted, it was often extremely difficult for doctors to give accurate predictions of how much time patients 'had left' and, for some patients at least, outliving the anticipated time of death could have devastating effects. To give an extreme illustration here, I encountered several patients who had asked their hospital consultant to predict how much time they had left to live and, on the basis of the consultant's estimation, they had opened their diaries and identified and planned for what they thought would be their exact day of death (we see a reason here why consultants are often very reluctant to answer such a question). Linda, for example, had been given a prognosis of around three months by her hospital doctor and, by the time she was admitted to the hospice, she was convinced that she only had a week left to live. During this week, she wrote letters to all of her friends and distant relatives to say her final farewells. The day before she expected to die, she summoned her son and two daughters to her bedside to distribute her jewellery and other personal possessions, together with final sentiments and words of advice (in a manner somewhat akin to a Hollywood deathbed scene). Despite staff's gentle warnings to the contrary, she remained convinced that she would die peacefully in her sleep that night. She was somewhat dismayed, therefore, when she woke up the following morning. Her despondency escalated as the days passed and visits from her children became increasingly stilted and awkward; neither party knew what to say to the other and the visits were pervaded by embarrassed silences. Linda did not die for a further three weeks. During the final week she was alive, she made several direct requests for euthanasia, claiming that she felt extremely angry and cheated. Linda, it would seem, had broken her connections with family and friends too prematurely, leaving her in the awkward and distressing situation of being 'socially dead' whilst still alive.

The experiences of patients who suffered from 'social death' bear some distinct parallels to the long-term suffering encountered by the Holocaust survivors studied by Langer (1996). Langer, in an attempt to understand why a number of survivors have recently requested that their bodies be buried at Birkenau, develops the idea of 'missed destiny', which he describes as being 'the condition of having missed one's intended destiny by surviving one's own death' (1996: 58). Many such survivors not only outlived their own families and friends; they had also survived 'the German intention to murder every living Jew with no exceptions' (ibid.). Consequently, as Langer further suggests, the long-term effects of the Holocaust had collapsed the conventional distinctions between living and dying, because those 'who outlived their doom' (1996: 62) were, nonetheless, 'plunged into a death-in-life milieu from which survival did not bring escape' (1996: 59). In a sense, then, the Holocaust survivors, like the hospice patients considered above, were cast into a state of liminality, because part of their self had become irretrievably lost at the time that the mass murder of the Jews took place.

One can also see some similarities between the experiences of hospice patients who 'lived too long' and the patients studied by Zussman in his observational research in two intensive care units in America. Zussman observed that doctors would generally only apply aggressive therapies in cases where they believed that a patient was capable of regaining a reasonable lifestyle. When doctors were pressed as to what they considered a reasonable lifestyle to be, the most common suggestion they made was that a patient should have a realistic chance of recovering sufficient mental clarity to be able to communicate and engage with family and friends in meaningful ways (1992: 129–30). In other words, a life was only considered to be worth living (and saving), so long as the potential to form and maintain interpersonal relations remained. Much the same observation has been made by McCormick who found that one of the main justifications medical professionals now give for not providing life-sustaining measures to anencephalic (brain-dead) infants is that they lack the potentiality to generate and sustain human relationships (1990: 33); in other words, they lack the capacity to become persons, in the sense defined in this study, and therefore to possess a full self. Indeed, all the examples presented here highlight the relational/exterior aspects of the self (see Chapter 1), a characteristic that seems to have been largely ignored in the literature cited in the previous two chapters, since it has focused more or less exclusively upon the development of the autonomous (embodied) components of 'Western' selfhood.

'Dying too soon': the 'special case' patient

Whilst many patients 'lived too long', others encountered the opposite problem: that of 'dying too soon'. Such patients were fully embedded within networks of relationships at the time they were admitted to the hospice, and, furthermore, were likely to 'pass away' before they and their family had adjusted to the idea of the 'loss' that their death would bring about. Several related factors distinguished these particular patients from the majority who received care within the hospice. First they were typically young people, often with young families; second, their prognosis had been very recent and unexpected; and, third, they had deteriorated extremely rapidly following the onset of terminal disease. As a consequence, there was often extremely limited time for the patient, and those in significant relationships with him or her, to prepare for, and to come to terms with, the impending death.

These particular patients – 'special case' patients as they were termed by hospice staff – were the ones for whom 'nothing is too much trouble' (Mark, hospice doctor). In practice this meant that the patient and his or her family were offered the full intervention and support of the multi-disciplinary team, and 'special case' patients often provoked extended, emotional discussions amongst staff in their hand-overs and multi-disciplinary team meetings. In addition to receiving counselling and other forms of psycho-social support, 'special case' patients often requested, and received, active medical interventions from staff such as blood transfusions and steroids. The aim of these interventions was to sustain a patient's strength and sentience (and thus their 'I can'; the embodied aspects of their selfhood) until the point they and their family members had prepared for the death. In practice, however, such attempts rarely 'bought' patients enough time; a phenomenon which had devastating effects upon all those involved.

Case study – Tony

Tony was a 45-year-old man who had lung cancer. He had been married twice and had a 6-year-old son, Joe, from his second marriage. He had only recently been informed of his diagnosis, and when I first spoke to him he claimed that both he and his wife were still 'numbed' by the shock of the news. The couple had recently moved house, and Tony was admitted to the hospice because he needed somewhere to stay for a week whilst their new home was being decorated.

A few days after his admission, Tony began to deteriorate extremely rapidly. He became very drowsy and he also developed problems with his breathing which caused him to suffer from sudden and violent attacks of coughing and choking. Whilst he had originally been admitted for respite care, it quickly became apparent to staff that he would need to remain in the hospice for terminal care. One of the doctors estimated that he might not live for more than a few days. At this stage, Tony and his wife were referred to the hospice counsellor. After an emotional meeting with the couple, the counsellor informed her colleagues that Tony and his wife had not yet told their son that he was going to die. Tony, although very tired and lethargic, felt strongly that he should break the news to Joe himself and suggested that the two of them should spend some time alone together. The couple also wanted Tony to be alert, sitting upright in bed, and ideally back at home, when he spoke to Joe.

The hospice doctors were thus left with the practical problem of 'perking' Tony up. They decided to reduce his morphine (which contributed to his drowsiness) and they also gave him a large dose of steroids which acted as a stimulus. The doctors recognised that the changes to his medication would only have a temporary effect, and warned the couple that they had very limited time to play around with. Because Tony was too unwell to return home for even a brief period, staff decided to move him into a side room, as this would give him more privacy to talk to Joe. Tony's wife arranged to bring Joe into the hospice to see his father the following day.

Whilst the changes to Tony's medication did have a brief stimulating effect, he deteriorated much faster than his doctors had hoped. During the night, he began to suffer from severe attacks of hyperventilation and pain which caused him to become extremely anxious. By the time I arrived at the hospice the following morning, the sound of his coughing and shouting could be heard throughout the building: Tony was writhing around in his bed, sweating, tossing and turning. Shortly afterwards, medical staff decided that they had no choice but to sedate him heavily. As one of the doctors pointed out at the time, Tony was no longer in any state to talk to his son, and it would be kinder to his family if he looked peaceful. Staff expressed considerable anguish that they had not been able to do more to help the family out earlier. Tony died that evening without getting a chance to say 'good-bye' to his son. During the afternoon, a nurse spent a couple of hours with Joe going through a chapter in a book designed to help a child come to terms with the death of a parent.

Tony's death was considered by his wife and staff alike to have been extremely harrowing. A death which takes a young person away from their family would almost certainly be considered tragic under any circumstances. In Tony's case, however, such a sense of tragedy was heightened because he did not have the opportunity to say 'good-bye' to the young son he was leaving behind.[1] Tony spent his last hours in considerable distress. Whilst staff did attempt to make him 'look peaceful' by sedating him heavily, his shouting and attacks of hyperventilation continued right up until the point at which he died. In their opinion, Tony's physical pain could not be successfully 'controlled' because he was dying leaving social and emotional concerns unresolved. Such a belief stemmed from their conception that a patient's 'total pain' experience involves a mutually affecting blend of physical, emotional, social and spiritual concerns; a conception which both reflects and reinforces a relational, intersubjective notion of the person/self (see Chapter 1).

Like most 'special case' patients, Tony later became the subject of a staff case conference, which was set up to enable members of the multi-disciplinary team to reflect upon their practices and explore ways in which 'things could have been done better'. It was a common complaint amongst staff in such meetings that they could actually do very little to help 'special case' patients, in large part because hospital consultants would rarely 'let go' of younger patients and would continue to apply aggressive curative therapies right up to the point at which they were close to death. As a result, many younger patients were only referred on to the hospice (if they were at all) within a matter of days or even hours of actually dying. 'Special case' patients, as staff further pointed out, had rarely prepared for death prior to their admission to the hospice because they had believed that, for as long as they were receiving aggressive therapies in hospital, there was continued hope of a cure.

As I have already indicated, all the 'special case' patients I encountered were comparatively young, the majority being in their thirties and forties.[2] Elderly patients rarely caused much of a ripple in the day-to-day working practices of the hospice, except on those distressing occasions when a patient became psychotic in one of the wards, or suffered from bodily unboundedness in an extreme form. It would be true to say that, as a general rule, older patients were more accepting of death than their younger counterparts: indeed, as I described earlier, some older patients appeared to actively welcome the prospect of death. It would seem, therefore, that this phenomenon can be explained by the fact that older patients – by virtue of their position in the life course – are more likely than their younger counterparts to lack a medium of sociality and reciprocity through which the self can be generated and expressed. As Hockey suggests:

> While individuals who die before the age of seventy may leave gaps – empty social roles, ruptured relationships, un-

finished business – those who survive the age of eighty may
find they have toppled over the edge of the social 'map'.

(Hockey 1990: 109)

Nevertheless, some older patients did have active and ongoing
relationships with family and friends and, as a consequence, they
also often had a strong will to continue to live. In private, a couple
of nurses expressed their cynicism that most members of staff
would only 'tear their hair out' in cases where there was a young
patient involved: in their opinion, ageism was latent within the
hospice and in society at large.

The 'making' and 'unmaking' of self through social connections

The above material thus indicates the importance of family and
other interpersonal relationships in contemporary English
conceptions of self. There is much therefore in these observations
that concords with Strathern's suggestion that, in the modern
English context, it is through relationships that the parties involved
are produced and reproduced as unique entities: a phenomenon
which leads her to argue that 'individuality' is 'both a fact of and
"after" kinship' (1992b: 15). As Strathern goes on to argue, modern
English 'individuals are not in themselves relations' (1992b: 78),
rather it is through one's locatedness within a constellation of
interpersonal ties that one's sense of self (as a unique entity) is
realised and sustained (ibid.). The implication of such an analytical
perspective is that, if one is removed from one's interpersonal
network, one's sense of self will be lost;[3] a situation which did
appear to occur amongst many of the patients with whom I
worked. Indeed, it has been rightly pointed out to me that – despite
the lack of detail in Tony's case study – this particular account
retains much more of a 'person present' sense about it than many
of the cases presented in this book. This could be explained by the
fact that Tony was one of the few patients I encountered in the
hospice who actually retained his self, through his close and
continued involvement with both his family and hospice staff, more
or less right up until the point at which he died.

The centrality of interpersonal relationships to contemporary
'Western' experiences and conceptions of self has also been
recognised and highlighted by other writers. Luckmann, for
example, has argued that 'familism' and 'sexuality' (1967: 106111)

have become central to 'the "autonomous" individual's quest for self-expression and self-realization' (1967: 111; see also Zaretsky 1976); a phenomenon which the disciplines of psychology and psychoanalysis both reflect and reinforce (Lasch 1977; Rose 1990). Similarly, Berger and Luckmann suggest that,

> significant others occupy a central position in the economy of reality maintenance. They are particularly important for the ongoing confirmation of that crucial element of reality we call identity. To retain confidence that he [sic] is indeed who he thinks he is, the individual requires not only implicit confirmation of this identity that even casual everyday contacts will supply, but the explicit and emotionally charged confirmation that his significant others bestow on him.
>
> (Berger and Luckmann 1971: 170)

Yet, it is in the work of Giddens (1991, 1993), that the most comprehensive description and analysis appears to reside. Giddens observes that the self is 'reflexively made' in the context of high or late modernity, and that the emergence of the 'pure relationship' has become central to this process. The pure relationship, he suggests, is entered into for its own sake, 'for what can be derived by each person from sustained association with another' (1993: 58), and is 'continued only in so far as it is thought by both parties to deliver enough satisfactions for each individual to stay within it' (ibid.). Whilst such a relationship is primarily dyadic in nature, a 'given individual is likely to be involved in several forms which tend towards the pure type' (1991: 97). Pure relationships, Giddens observes, have not only come into existence in the domains of sexuality, marriage and friendship; as he further points out, 'the more a child moves toward adulthood and autonomy', the more elements of the pure relationship also come into play within this particular interpersonal arena (1991: 98, 1993: 188).[4]

Whilst writers such as Berger and Luckmann have tended to explain the rising importance of intimate relationships as being a defence against the enveloping outside world – as a 'haven in a heartless world' (Lasch 1977) – Giddens develops a more broad and overarching perspective. In opposition to the idea that the quest for a source of 'ultimate significance' is a universal human need, albeit one which is increasingly confined within the private sphere of home and family (Luckmann 1967; Zaretsky 1976), Giddens argues that the 'need' is itself a product of culturally constructed norms and ideologies. As he suggests, pure relationships are 'thoroughly permeated by mediated influences coming from large-scale social systems, and usually actively organise those influences within the sphere of such relationships' (1991: 7). The values of 'autonomy' and 'individuality' so prized within contemporary 'Western' contexts are realised through pure relationships, precisely because these relationships are entered into as a matter of choice. One's sense of personal 'uniqueness', then, is expressed and achieved in the setting of high modernity by having an array of 'unique' others to reflect and affirm one's 'individuality'.

Giddens' analysis represents a significant advance on earlier studies but, in spite of this, there are some difficulties with his approach. As writers such as Shilling and Mellor (1996) have pointed out, there is a certain naive idealism embedded within his notion of the pure relationship. One needs only to look at Skeggs' (1997) study of contemporary working-class women, for example, to recognise that marriages (amongst members of the working classes at least) are often entered into for practical and financial reasons; love and romance may not be the sole or even the major motives. One could also argue that relationships are often not as easily terminated as Giddens' analysis suggests; couples staying together for 'the benefit of the children' being good cases in point. Yet whilst critical attention has focused most centrally upon Giddens' approach in this regard, concern is also increasingly being directed towards his seemingly 'disembodied' conception of the pure relationship.[5] As Shilling and Mellor (citing the work of Jary and Jary (1995)) point out, 'Giddens' analysis is predicated on the view that intimacy is above all a matter of emotional *communication* with oneself and others' (1996: 9, original emphasis), with the consequence that 'he marginalizes the more sensual or carnal dimensions of both close relationships and of those moral concerns that characterize people's lives' (1996: 13). Hence they urge that more attention be paid 'to the "underbelly" of modernity' (ibid.).

Indeed, it is largely in response to such 'disembodied' analyses of emotions and relationships, that a revival of interest in the work of the symbolic interactionist Erving Goffman is taking place (for example, Turner 1992; Shilling 1993; Crossley 1995; Seymour 1998; Williams and Bendelow 1998). In his various studies such as *The Presentation of Self in Everyday Life* (1959), *Relations in Public* (1962) and *Stigma* (1963), Goffman highlights the various ways in which the appearance and presentation of the body affect and mediate micro-social interactions. In their day-to-day interactions, 'actors', he suggests, constantly 'give off' and receive bodily information, and it is on the basis of such information that social encounters are framed and proceed. Goffman's work thus provides a springboard for bringing the body into the picture, but it is worth recognising that his analysis is predicated primarily upon the notion of the 'performative' body; that is, of the body of 'appearance, display and impression management' discussed at the start of Chapter 3. It is for this reason, as I now highlight, that even the most liberal readings of his work can only partly incorporate the body into studies of relationships and intimacy.

Whilst the ethnographic material outlined thus far in this chapter has focused upon the loss of self that occurs following a loss of interpersonal relationships, a patient's bodily deterioration can also often be implicated in the processes which lead to his or her social death. In other words, there are indeed strong grounds for arguing that relationships cannot be considered separately from bodies in either practical or analytical terms: as Seymour observes, the body is in fact 'critical to the development of social routines and relationships' (1998: 51). In this regard, the 'performative' aspects of embodiment are certainly important to the formation, maintenance and loss of social and emotional ties. Such a phenomenon becomes only too apparent when the experiences of patients who underwent rapid and often very distressing changes in their physical *appearance* are explored. Kerry, for example, was a woman in her thirties whose husband of three years had not only stopped showing her any signs of affection, 'it's even got to the stage where he can't stand being in the same room as me'. Kerry's bodily appearance had altered radically following the onset of her illness: she had had a double mastectomy and was still bald following her most recent course of chemotherapy; her legs and arms were extremely swollen and bloated; and her cancer had spread so rapidly and aggressively that tumours had begun to protrude through her back and other parts of her body. She fully understood why her husband 'now finds me totally repulsive'. The Goffman-esque notion of 'stigma', leading to the avoidance of the patient by others, is very evident in this and other examples (see, for example, p. 45).

Yet, as I indicated above, to focus solely upon the 'performative' body of 'appearance' and 'display' presents only a partial picture: other aspects of embodiment are equally, if not more, central to the 'making' and 'unmaking' of self through social connectivity. As my observations in earlier chapters can be used to highlight, bodily mobility also underlies the processes by which social contacts are made and/or sustained; a situation made especially evident in the case of patients who, after losing their mobility, found themselves increasingly physically isolated from others. This phenomenon was movingly highlighted by Fred whose experiences were described in Chapter 2. After Fred had lost his ability to walk, he ceased to be able to go to his local pub and pensioners' club where he had previously met and made new friends. Instead, he found himself confined within his own home, feeling like 'an animal trapped in a cage', with only brief visits from a care assistant and a neighbour. Robillard, in his auto-ethnographic account of having severe muscular dystrophy, likewise draws our attention to the difficulties of interacting with others while wheelchair-bound and (in his case) unable to move his head and upper body at will. In his study he points to the various difficulties (and sense of anger) he experienced whilst attending a party where he was left in his wheelchair amongst a group of people he did not particularly know (or wish to get to know). He was neither able move himself to the people with whom he actually wanted to socialise, nor was he even able to turn his head so that he could, at the very least, attract their attention (1996: 23–5). Seymour, in her research on men and women with profound bodily paralysis, similarly observes that her informants' inability 'to spontaneously translate emotions into conventionally recognised acts of endearment' such as touching, cuddling and hugging, often led to an erosion of their interpersonal relationships (1998: 75).

Yet mobility is not the only aspect of bodily autonomy that underlies and underwrites the processes by which interpersonal relationships are forged between self and others. As the material discussed in the previous chapter highlights, bodily boundedness is also critical both to one's own conception of self, and to sustaining the self through relationships with others. Indeed, we have seen a number of examples in which patients encountered the harrowing situation of being left alone by family and friends after the boundaries of their bodies fell severely and irreversibly apart. Even those closest to a patient often found themselves repelled, quite literally, by the smells and substances which oozed and seeped from his or her porous body. Patients, as a consequence, were often left in a situation of extreme social isolation.

Giddens' approach to the 'pure relationship' thus is somewhat unidimensional and simplistic, for we have seen a number of complex ways in which a patient's body may also interweave with, and impinge upon, his or her relationships with family, friends and others (of which bodily 'performance' is only one aspect). Nonetheless, a number of elements in Giddens' analysis do remain both helpful and relevant, most notably the emphasis he places upon the autonomous component of the pure relationship as being a central means by which one's 'individuality' is reflected and reinforced. Certainly, a number of examples can be drawn from Chapter 4 which indicate that it is not in fact enough to be embedded in a network of family and friends: the relationships between patient and others must themselves be based upon a certain level of *mutual autonomy*. Indeed, we have seen that, when a family member provides a 'high-dependency' patient with 'hands-on care', neither party in this particular relationship experiences a reinforcement of their own 'individuality'. To the contrary, the carer's body and self become entwined with the body of the patient. It could be further suggested here that, when a family member or friend becomes a patient's carer, the relationship between the two parties often ceases to be of 'pure type', since many carers often have little, or no choice, over whether they take on the responsibility for providing a patient with 'hands-on' care (patients, likewise, exercise little choice over who actually cares for them). Certainly, it has been recognised within the academic literature that the very label 'carer' is not incidental but, rather, ideologically loaded. As Brotchie and Hills observe, the very word 'carer' transforms the 'caring role' into an obligation rather than a choice, because to chose not to take on the responsibilities associated with such a role can easily be equated with 'not being caring' (1991: 34). Hence there is a strong moral obligation placed upon patients' relatives to provide them with unpaid, cost-effective care, often within their own homes (ibid.).

Whilst Giddens' concept of autonomy is salient it is, needless to say, essentially premised upon the 'mental' conception of the 'freedom to chose'; therefore, the *bodily* components of autonomy also need to be more explicitly recognised and underscored within such an analytical approach. Autonomy, in this latter sense, not only involves being able to bodily enact one's own wishes and intentions, but also to maintain control of the physical boundaries of one's own body.

Disintegrating selves: where do gender and class fit in?

Degenderisation

As I indicated in Chapter 1, gender has not featured prominently in the main sections of this book for reasons that are largely pragmatic: gendered differences were not generally marked amongst the patients with whom I worked. Male and female patients encountered similar problems with social isolation; the effects of bodily deterioration, likewise, eroded and undermined their sense of self in the same ways (high-dependency patients, for example, used the same metaphors to describe themselves irrespective of whether they were men or women). Patients also often ceased to respond to their situations in stereotypically gendered ways: few tears were shed in the final stages approaching death; masculine bravado and jocularity were equally absent.[6] This latter observation is in fact crucial, for on close scrutiny it appears that one of the principal reasons why gendered differences were not prominent in this study is because patients often experienced a disinvestment of their 'masculinity' or 'femininity' even in the early stages of their illness and deterioration.

It is noteworthy that when patients (both in day care and the hospice) did make direct (and unprompted) references to gendered aspects of their sense of self, they did so only to indicate or berate a sense of loss that had already occurred. Recall, for example, the interview I conducted with Jan whilst she was attending day care. After Jan had had a double mastectomy, she said that she found it extremely difficult to see herself as a woman or to contemplate the possibility of having an intimate relationship with a partner (see p. 45). Similarly, Hazel, 32, who had cancer of the cervix and had lost most of her hair following a recent course of palliative chemotherapy, offered the following comment when she reflected upon the impact of her illness upon her life:

> It does affect your femininity a lot. I mean, I don't look at clothes anymore. I don't look at makeup. I don't even look in the mirror if I can avoid it. I had some passport photos done and I was so shocked by my appearance. I just tore them up.

Another day care patient, Ron, pointed to his own feelings of 'degenderisation' after he developed cancer of the prostate and spinal secondaries which caused him to become paralysed from the waist downwards and thus (as he pointed out) impotent:

> My illness has made me feel very humble. It's made me less of a man I suppose. ... Nurses come round twice a day to help wash and dress me. I don't care if there's anyone else in the room, even if they're cleaning my penis at the time.

Ron went on to tell me that he and his wife started 'sleeping in separate beds' after he became unwell. I was also informed by Ron's Macmillan nurse that his wife had recently complained that she did not have 'a man anymore'.

To understand patients' experiences of 'degenderisation' it is first necessary to explore the complex processes by which gender is constructed and evaluated to start with. As West and Zimmerman highlight, 'gender is not simply an aspect of what one is, but, more fundamentally, it is something that one *does*, and does recurrently in interaction with others' (1987: 140, original emphasis). Gender, in other words, is not an innate category or experience, but 'a situated doing carried out in the virtual or real presence of others who are presumed to be oriented to its production' (1987: 126). As Butler, in a related fashion, suggests, gender is not something with which one is born, it is a process, a becoming, achieved through 'the repeated stylization of the body, a set of repeated acts within a highly rigid regulatory frame that congeal over time to produce the appearance of substance, of a natural sort of being' (1990: 33; see also Butler 1993; Connell 1993, 1995). Such conceptions of gender are extremely illuminating: if gender is something that has to be *continuously* performed in everyday interactions, the implication is that, when either the body that is supposed to go with that performance, or the social web itself, begin to be lost, so too will one's gender.[7]

Certainly, a key theme of observation in this chapter has been the various ways in which patients can, and do become disembedded from their social networks prior to death. Patients, in other words, often lost those relationships (real and/or anticipated) through which their gender could be interactively reflected and affirmed (indeed, Jan's sense of loss of her womanhood makes no sense outside her conception that other people had also ceased to see her in that way). And part of this loss of sociality (and hence gender) could also be understood as stemming from the fact that many patients had lost those aspects of their bodies necessary to 'do' gender to start with: body parts associated with sexuality and sexual functioning. Such a phenomenon is clearly alluded to in Jan's and Ron's comments above. It has also been observed by other researchers who have worked with patients who have cancer. Cannon (1988), for example, in her study of women with breast cancer, found that a significant proportion mourned 'the loss of their femininity,' particularly after one or both breasts had to be amputated. Gordon, in his study of men with testicular cancer, likewise noticed that it was not uncommon for these men to report that they felt 'less masculine' immediately after surgery and chemotherapy because they were unable to function normally sexually (1995: 252; see also Sontag 1991: 18).[8]

The elision between gender and sexuality is so seamless here, and so thoroughly embedded within 'Western' constructions, that it appears hardly worth noting. However, as many analysts of modern 'Western' gender and sexuality have suggested (e.g. Green 1997; Ariès and Bèjin 1985; Butler 1990, 1993; Weeks 1986; Caplan 1987; Laqueur 1992), it is the historical development of this elision which lies at the heart of most people's daily experience of gender. This is especially important in terms of its implications for people's sense of self in the modern 'Western' context. Here, to lose one's 'sex' is to lose both gender and sexuality simultaneously, for the one implies the other inexorably. But it is also much more than this; it is to lose a central part of who one is in the world *vis-à-vis* others. It is this aspect of gender loss, the loss of one's embeddedness within social networks, that patients were referring to when they expressed regret about the attrition of certain sexual bodily capacities and characteristics.

The class paradox

It might seem somewhat paradoxical that, despite the disintegration of self that patients underwent, many appeared to retain their class attributes and tastes more or less right up to the point at which they finally died. Such a phenomenon, as I suggested in Chapter 1, became particularly noticeable in the ways in which space was appropriated and used within the hospice setting. Although the hospice was designed to accommodate the majority of its patients in wards, the building did contain some side rooms. When these side rooms were not being occupied by confused patients (see Chapter 4) or those with severely unbounded bodies (see Chapter 5) they were almost always allocated to middle-class patients. Since the hospice did not admit private patients, side rooms were not assigned on the basis of who could afford to pay for them. Side rooms, it should be further noted, afforded certain luxuries not available to patients in wards: most had en-suite toilets and bathrooms and all contained items such as remote controlled television sets. Side rooms also had doors which could be closed, allowing patients more privacy to talk to family and friends, or to shut people out.

Interestingly, most patients had strong views about their preferred choice of location within the hospice, and such views appeared to be rooted in class-based tastes. Working-class patients often said that they valued being in a ward because 'you get all the attention here'. Patients often followed such a comment with the claim that they would feel 'scared' and 'lonely' if they were placed in a room on their own. Middle-class patients, in contrast, often appeared to hold a very different set of values: for them the privacy and the comfort afforded by side rooms was very important. Middle-class patients also made it clear that they did not want to 'muck in' with working-class patients in wards and other communal areas within the hospice building. As a former newspaper editor suggested, 'in a ward ... it all becomes far too superficial ... it's as if they honestly believe that by clinging together, by safety in numbers, the problem will go away'. Another middle-class patient, Marilyn, pointed to the 'awful experiences' she had had during previous hospital stays (when she was receiving curative therapies) to explain why she appreciated being given a side room in the hospice: 'the other patients [in the wards] used to drive me mad ... all their menial conversations and inane questions. ... Frankly, I'm much happier on my own.'

To understand why patients retained their class-based preferences and tastes, even after so much of their capacity to see themselves, and to be seen, as persons had gone, the observations developed earlier on in this chapter are relevant. As the experiences of 'special case' patients have usefully illustrated, selfhood is not necessarily, and always, dictated by bodily states: 'special case' patients had their selves preserved from 'without'; in this particular case through other people who continued to engage and interact with them.[9] One could thus see the retention of class attributes as being a further exemplar of this process of preservation of self from 'without'. To develop such a perspective the work of Bourdieu is helpful, most particularly his notion of *habitus*. For Bourdieu, habitus is an 'acquired system of generative positions' (1977: 95); a socially and historically determined 'structuring structure' which mediates between human actions on the one hand and a wider 'social system' on the other. Habitus, for Bourdieu, inculcates particular mind-sets and patterns of taste which provide 'social actors' with class-dependent, pre-disposed, yet seemingly 'naturalised' ways of thinking, acting and being (1984: 170). As such, it serves as a means by which social distinctions based on class (and indeed the social classes themselves) are produced and reproduced within a society over time. Whilst Bourdieu has been charged with remaining trapped within an objectivist position which largely strips agency of its critical reflexive character (Jenkins 1992; Williams 1995), his work, as Williams points out, does serve as a necessary corrective to the view that lifestyles are simply a matter of choice within a society supposedly characterised by a growth in social reflexivity (1995: 588, 592).

Within the hospice it was notable that staff, as a matter of routine, tried to accommodate patients in wards or side rooms according to their previous occupational status. Middle-class patients were, whenever possible, admitted to the privacy of side rooms, whereas working-class patients invariably found themselves allocated to beds in wards. One side room in the hospice was in fact informally named the 'VIP suite'; a term which meant, in practice, that the room was earmarked for members of professional classes. One could thus reasonably argue that the architectural design of the hospice, coupled with the working practices of staff, fostered an environment, a 'habitus', within which the class-based attributes of patients could be, and indeed often were, preserved.

This chapter, then, has been concerned with sociality; that is, with different forms of social relationships and the different ways in which people become embedded within, and disembedded from, social networks. Some aspects of this phenomenon are crucially related to embodiment (e.g. gender), whereas others are more external and relational (e.g. class). Nonetheless, what this chapter has brought out very clearly is how central the interplay between social networks, embodiment and social interactions (including spaces for interaction) is to the performance and maintenance of the self. This has been possible by looking at the complex and diverse ways in which the exterior aspects of selfhood (interpersonal relationships) are lost, sometimes gradually, and sometimes very suddenly, amongst patients who are dying.

6

FINAL REFLECTIONS

I don't like the idea of lingering. If it's going to happen let it happen; not all this hanging on dying inch by inch, fighting every scrap of the way.

(Ann, hospice patient)

I would have liked a quicker exit, a sudden heart attack I suppose.

(Ron, hospice patient)

Dying as a phase of liminality in modern 'Western' contexts

Many modern 'Western' people, as Hinton suggests, 'say it is not so much death as dying that they fear' (1967: 23),[1] an observation that has been echoed by Weisman (1979: 69–70) and Backer (1982: 23). Such a phenomenon, it is argued, is comparatively recent: as Kearl observes, it is only over the past two centuries that expressed fears have shifted away from post-mortem concerns (e.g. judgement, Hell and reincarnation) to centre more exclusively upon anxieties surrounding the dying process itself (1989: 14). Certainly, as the quotes above suggest, many of the patients in this study became extremely distressed about the lingering ways in which they were dying. When patients reflected upon their own experiences, and those of other patients around them, it is very noteworthy that a large number spoke of wishing that they had died suddenly of a heart attack. Whilst the prospect of death could be extremely upsetting to patients, the experience of a drawn-out period of dependency, decline and social disengagement prior to death often seemed to provoke even greater distress.

171

The patients discussed in this book are not alone in this regard: during the past five or so years, there has been an explosion of debates within the media and academia that centre upon subjects such as physician-assisted suicide, living wills[2] and a patient's 'right to die'. The recent deluge of articles, documentaries and books now addressing these issues has prompted academics such as Walter to argue that: 'All this sounds like a society obsessed with death, not one that denies it' (1994: 1). Yet, as the observations developed in previous pages suggest, what is actually being reflected upon in academic and media discourses, and indeed amongst patients with debilitating illnesses themselves, is not so much the topic of death *per se*, but the question of what makes a person a *person*, and at what stage in one's illness and deterioration attributes of person/self are so irretrievably lost that death seems a preferable option to life. Suffering, in this sense, can be closely connected to a poor 'quality of life', since a poor 'quality of life' occurs when some or all of the 'potentialities for personhood' are absent (Callahan 1990: 250).[3]

These kinds of debates have almost certainly been stimulated by advances in acute care medicine which, as Callahan observes, have been so successful in sustaining and lengthening life, that some lives are now being preserved at the expense of their quality (1987, 1990). Indeed, as Gerhardt (1990) points out, 'quality of life' has only become an issue of medical importance in the last forty years or so, and, for him, can be connected to two related accomplishments of clinical practice: first, that infectious diseases (e.g. pneumonia, influenza), which were major causes of death of the chronically ill until the 1940s, can now often be successfully cured; second, that dramatic improvements in drug treatments and surgical interventions have radically improved the life expectancy of diabetics, cancer patients, epileptics, patients with MS and others. Consequently, many people are now living for longer, but often in a chronic state of ill health (Callahan 1987: 20; Walter and Shannon 1990: 107). As Lofland observes, a new element of the dying situation in the modern 'medicalised' 'West' is that dying itself is often highly prolonged (1978: 18).

Yet whilst advances in medicine and technology can be used to explain why the occurrence of long, protracted periods of chronic illness have become much more common in modern 'Western' contexts (and indeed in other parts of the world such as Asia where 'Western' healthcare provision and social patterns are increasingly taking hold), one must look to broader cultural factors to understand why the experience of a prolonged period of deterioration and decline prior to death is seen, and experienced, in 'self-debasing' ways. As the following discussions highlight, the pre-mortem disintegration of self experienced by many of the patients in this book is not a universal, self-evident process, but one that can be connected to the modern 'Western' conception that death itself is now seen as final, marking an *irreversible cessation* in the existence of a societal member (see Backer 1982). Indeed, in cultural settings where death is conceived more as a transitory phase leading to another form of existence, a reversal may occur wherein the disinvestment and loss of personhood occurs *after* the point understood as death in modern 'Western' contexts.

The modern 'Western' understanding of death, it is argued, has developed in tandem with an ideology of 'individualism'; that is with the conception that societal members now compete with one another on an equal footing, and status is achieved rather than given by virtue of descent (see La Fontaine 1985: 133–9).[4] As Bloch and Parry suggest, the idea of death as a 'terminus' has arisen because it serves to reinforce 'our' belief that persons are unique entities with distinct and unrepeatable biographies (1982: 15): hence a similar conception of death can also be found in other types of society where 'individuality' is marked (see, for example, Woodburn's (1982) discussion of death beliefs and practices amongst so called 'immediate-return' hunter-gatherer societies such as the Hadza of Northern Tanzania and the Mbuti Pygmies of Zaire). In contrast, in cultural contexts which approximate more closely to Dumont's (1985, 1986) notion of a 'holistic' type (see Chapter 1), death may be conceived instead as a phase of transition – a phenomenon that has been pointed to by writers such as Hertz (1960), and later by Huntington and Metcalf (1980) and Danforth (1982), in their studies of double funeral practices. As Hertz observes in his study of funerals in Malayo-Polynesian societies, the first burial, involving a temporary disposal of the corpse, represents a process of disaggregation, and the second a process of 'rebirth' or reinstallation (1960).

The conception that death is part of a continual cycle of renewal rather than an individual extinction, as Bloch and Parry (1982) argue, serves an important ideological function in reifying and reproducing social groups based on ascriptive statuses. In such societies, legitimacy, they suggest, is derived by stressing continuity between generations, in particular through the notion of descent. The death of a 'role occupant', which by its very nature implies discontinuity, thus represents an ideological challenge to the system's legitimacy. This problem, they observe, is overcome in a number of societies by underplaying 'individuality' and individual mortality through symbolically equating birth with death. The underemphasis of the 'individual' serves to enforce the belief that the essence of the person belongs to the wider social group, not simply to the body she or he inhabits (1982: 11). Consequently, in clan-based societies, individual members are perceived as a recyclable part of the wider social group (see, for example, Bloch 1986: 168; Bloch and Parry 1982: 8), whereas, for example, in Hindu contexts, the death of the person is believed to regenerate the entire cosmic order (Parry 1982).[5]

Whilst it is unwise to posit too sharp a distinction between 'holistic' and 'individualistic' societies (see Morris 1994; Bloch 1988),[6] such a distinction does allow some interesting points of comparison to be drawn. If one accepts that, in societies veering towards a 'holistic' type, death is often seen not as total annihilation, but rather (in some senses at least) as a phase of liminality (Danforth 1982: 37; Turner 1967), it follows that in 'individualistic' contexts where death is perceived as final, it is the process of dying which constitutes the liminal period. 'Individuals' in a state of liminality, as both Van Gennep (1972) and Douglas (1984) have forcefully argued, are regarded as vulnerable, polluting and dangerous because their 'betwixt and between' position leads to their status *as persons* becoming highly ambiguous. Hence it is possible to understand why it is dying rather than death that provokes greatest fear and anxiety in settings such as contemporary England; in particular a protracted period of deterioration and decline, since this constitutes an extended period of liminality.

Observations such as these also allow some noteworthy parallels (albeit simplistic) to be drawn between the experiences of dying patients in settings such as contemporary England, and 'post-mortem' experiences in more 'holistic' cultures such as India. In his study of cremation practices in Banaras, Parry, for example, describes how, prior to the cremation, the 'corpse' is believed to retain some of the 'life-force' and 'essence' of the person (1994: 181). It is only after the body is placed on the funeral pyre and the skull is broken that life is believed to be finally extinguished and death pollution begins (ibid.). Such an observation helps to explain why it is the corpse itself which is believed to be 'pre-eminently polluting and dangerous' (1994: 180), as well as constituting a source of sacredness (ibid.). Watson, in his study of Chinese mortuary rituals, similarly points to an 'extreme ambivalence shown towards the physical remains of the deceased' (1982: 155). The living can only access and use the bones of their ancestors after the flesh of the corpse has disintegrated completely (1982: 156), because the disintegration of the flesh is believed to occur at the same time as the 'setting of the spirit' (1982: 180). Clearly then, whilst in the modern English context the 'disintegration' of the person/self is intimately bound up with the deterioration and decline of the 'mortal', 'living flesh' and hence may precede death itself, in cultures where death is perceived more as a transitory phase, personhood, to some extent, dissipates *after* the point perceived as physical cessation in modern 'Western' settings.

These observations, furthermore, lend deep insights into why the body has been so central to the observations and analyses developed in this book. One can now see strong grounds for arguing that personhood has become particularly entwined with the body and bodily capacity in contexts such as modern England because, in a setting where death is thought of as final, the body has come to be perceived 'as a secularised private domain of the individual person' (Kleinman 1988: 11), rather than as 'a transitory vehicle, a means to higher spiritual ends' (Featherstone 1993: 186).[7] Hence Shilling's argument that, in a sense, modern 'Western' persons *are* their bodies; the body, he suggests, has become ever more important as 'constitutive of the self' (1993: 3). In such a setting, the disintegrating, decaying (but living body) may thus lead to a 'deconstitution' of self.

Since so much of patients' suffering – their disintegration of self – was manifest and experienced in pre-mortem, 'this-worldly' ways, it is perhaps not too surprising that religious beliefs rarely had a bearing on the ways in which patients tried to come to terms with their illness and deterioration. Religious belief, as Feifel observes, is commonly thought to serve as a 'major way of coping with the fear of death' (1974: 353, 1959). Yet for the patients involved in this study it was not really death as such that was the problem: it was dying. It is almost certainly for this reason that I did not notice any obvious differences between patients who claimed to be religious and those who did not.[8] Feifel, in his study of terminally ill patients likewise found that: 'Personal nearness to death ... did not reveal any differences between believers and unbelievers' (1974: 353); an observation further echoed by Kübler-Ross (1969: 237), Hinton (1967: 84) and Weisman (1979: 78ff.). I did not, furthermore, witness any last minute religious conversions in the hospice; a situation which was confirmed by the hospice chaplain when I interviewed her. In fact, if anything, the very distressing ways in which some patients deteriorated and rotted away within the hospice, prompted a small but significant minority of hitherto religious patients to question their faith, and sometimes to abandon it altogether. One bed-bound and doubly-incontinent patient, Alan, a man in his seventies, suggested that his belief in God had become 'much more lukewarm' in his later years. However, it had been his contact with patients in the hospice 'dying in such distress', which had particularly cast his beliefs into doubt. Another woman, Christine, threw her Bible out of her locker (quite literally), claiming that she could no longer believe in God after, 'seeing so much suffering around me'. Four women had died in her ward, one of whom became very paranoid and distressed and required heavy sedation (prior to being sedated, this particular woman had accused both staff and patients of being members of the IRA, and claimed that they were deliberately plotting to kill her). Christine herself suffered from chronic diarrhoea, causing perpetual problems with smell. It is very significant that she went on to liken her experience to 'the nearest thing I can imagine to *hell on earth*' (emphasis added); the 'this-worldliness' of her own and other patients' suffering was only too apparent.

It is, nonetheless, important to be reflexive about the specific nature of the hospice environment. As the observations developed in Chapter 4 highlighted, there are strong grounds for arguing that the hospice had become a 'sequestered space' for particularly distressing cases, especially for those involving extreme bodily disintegration and decay.

Palliative care: some implications of this study

Dear Julia,

I was encouraged to talk to you by [X]. I am a student who attended your lecture on hospice care. I was just telling [X] about the very optimistic experience I had when visiting [name of hospice omitted].

Anyway, I am talking from a relative's perspective as my husband's father is dying of cancer and is in there for medication control at the moment. The difference in approach from the hospital was amazing! Now, I know that there are reasons for hospitals not being equipped to deal with everything, and I am not judging, merely noticing. In the hospital we had in vain tried to talk to a nurse to get information re: medication, length of stay etc. My father-in-law seemed not to know what was going on apart from that he was in pain, and the tablets weren't helping (and he is not generally confused). No one could tell us anything and he left the hospital the same as he had come in. When he returned a week later because the pain was so bad, they referred him to [the hospice]. We went to see him there the other day. He was much calmer, just by knowing that if he asked, they would give him pain relief. When my husband asked about the length of his stay, a nurse came and sat with us all to explain what they were doing, why they were doing it, was there anything else we wanted done etc. My father-in-law now knows exactly how they're trying to help him and my husband also knows. I really felt that we were treated as people with our own lives etc. The whole atmosphere was calm, reassuring and ... well human!

I don't mean to say that you don't realise this, but after your lecture I felt a bit disillusioned about hospices. Now, I know you didn't mean they were all like that, or that they didn't still play a useful role, but I just thought I'd tell you of my very positive experience. Now, in fact my father-in-law will probably be one of these patients who will end up with an unbounded body as he has mouth and face cancer. He will most likely be suffering from bad odours as well. I think that we should all be concerned that the hospice movement should not end up as a dumping ground for unsavoury patients and I think your work is incredibly important to highlight this risk. As I see it, the good that the hospices can achieve is immense and I would not like it to change.

I hope you don't mind me writing to you about this. As I said, it is not to argue against your view, just to offer a bit of hopeful light! Anyway, I can always blame [X], since she told me to write!

Thank you for listening, and good luck with your work!
Yours sincerely,
[name omitted here][9]

This message was send to me by a medical student whose father-in-law, as it turns out, received care in the same hospice as I conducted my research (the author, I should say, was not aware of this fact). I have included it here because it puts across a point of view with which I am in total agreement: it has never been my intention to give the impression that hospices are simply 'doom and gloom places', nor for that matter that palliative care has nothing positive to offer to patients and their families and friends. The man whose experiences are described above clearly benefited both from the staff's willingness to talk to and spend time with him and his family, and from the excellent pain relief that was made available to him. One can, however, only speculate about his later experiences, as indeed the author of the message appears to do.

Certainly, few would disagree that, through the methods of pain control which were pioneered by Cicely Saunders, the modern hospice movement has made a very significant contribution to the alleviation of patients' suffering and distress. Few patients need now die in intense pain, and in the vast majority of cases, pain can either be completely, or at least partially relieved. Yet, as the material discussed in this book has vividly highlighted, the suffering that dying (and other) patients may endure is far broader than the experience of pain: suffering also involves the humiliation of physical dependence, loss of continence, and the distress of ceasing to be able to engage in meaningful relationships with others (see also Seale 1998; Caplan 1997). It is these latter components of suffering, sadly, that are not so easily or readily addressed by palliative systems of health care delivery.

Indeed, this book could be read at its core as a powerful critique of the modern hospice movement's aim of enabling patients to 'live until they die'. As I described in Chapter 1, the movement set itself the goal of pushing back a patient's social death to the point of physical death, through the belief that it is possible 'to maintain a patient's self-worth by demonstrating through sensitive and compassionate care that he or she is still of value to society' (National Council for Hospice and Specialist Palliative Care Services 1993: 14). Yet, as the observations developed in this book suggest, such a belief, however well intended, rests somewhat problematically upon a *disembodied* conception of the dying patient.[10] The idea that it is possible to 'die with dignity', regrettably, is thrown into doubt when what I have termed the 'bodily realities of dying' are explicitly recognised: a patient's bodily deterioration may have a 'non-negotiable', debasing impact upon his or her sense of self, and also upon his or her ability to sustain relationships with family and friends. In fact, Seale and Addington-Hall (1995) have made the somewhat ironic observation that patients who receive hospice care are more likely than other patients with similar physical and mental conditions to express the view that it would have been better if they had died earlier. As they suggest, good care, such as that offered by a hospice, might serve to increase patients' feelings of lost autonomy by reminding them of their declining ability to do things for themselves (1995: 587).

Findings such as these warn against complacency: we cannot assume that the modern hospice movement has had the radical effects that its pioneers intended. As Jennings argues in his recent critique of the ethics of hospice and palliative care, we can no longer afford to regard the movement's commitments as 'self-evident, noncontroversial, and in need of little explicit analysis and examination' (1997: 2). On the contrary, there is an urgent need for a more rigorous analysis of such taken-for-granted tenets as 'the prevention and relief of suffering', 'death with dignity' and 'the good death' (ibid.). Certainly, when tenets such as these are critically examined in the context of one of the most ethically contentious issues of our time – debates on euthanasia – the modern hospice movement's position becomes more problematic than many people would like to assume.

It hardly needs to be stated that proponents of hospice and palliative care are fundamentally opposed to euthanasia. We are told that, with the sensitive and compassionate care that palliative care professionals can now provide, there is no reason for patients to suffer and, if there is no reason for patients to suffer, it follows that there is also no need for patients to wish to have their deaths hastened (see, for example, Saunders 1993b; Cassidy 1994). Palliative care is thus commonly presented as the antidote to debates which centre upon thorny issues such as physician-assisted suicide and a patient's 'right to die'. Proponents of palliative care, needless to say, have not been immune to criticism in this and other related respects. As I indicated in Chapter 4, concern has recently been expressed about the equity of access to hospices and other palliative care services. Palliative care is principally geared towards patients with incurable cancer, which means that substantial numbers of other patients with chronic and debilitating conditions are excluded from these supposedly 'Rolls Royce' services (Clark and Seymour 1999). Additional concern, as I highlighted in Chapter 1, has focused upon the effects of the assimilation of the modern hospice movement into mainstream systems of biomedicine, most notably the supposed 'routinisation' that can occur (James 1986, 1994). The matter, however, does not stop here: it is the terms by which hospice and palliative care professionals voice their opposition to euthanasia that are starting to be subjected to critical attention. As both Seale (1998) and Caplan (1997) have recently pointed out, proponents of the modern hospice movement have to date made any discussion of assistance in dying off limits, on the grounds that it was – and is – unrelieved pain that prompts patients to wish to have their deaths hastened. Such a view, as Seale observes, is only too apparent in Cicely Saunders' suggestion that:

> 'Kill me,' a definite request for medically assisted suicide, though heard more often than it was 30 years ago, is still extremely uncommon. It may be voiced because of long unrelieved pain and is likely to fade away once this has been addressed as in almost all cases it can be.
>
> (Saunders 1992: 2, cited in Seale 1998: 185)

It is also echoed in a 1993 paper presented to the House of Lords Select Committee on Medical Ethics, in which the National Council for Hospice and Specialist Palliative Care Services presented its objections to the possible legalisation of euthanasia within the UK in the following terms:

> Too often patients and their relatives, and sometimes even their professional advisers, believe that terminal illness and great suffering inevitably and inexorably go hand in hand. With modern palliative methods almost all pain can be relieved, and can always be reduced. ... The killing of a patient in pain destroys the problem but does nothing to advance knowledge or to relieve the next sufferer.
>
> (National Council for Hospice and Specialist Palliative Care Services 1993: 14)

Yet, the close – and seemingly exclusive – relationship that is posited between 'suffering' and 'pain' is extremely problematic because suffering, as we have seen, is far broader than pain. One could actually take a slightly cynical stance here and suggest that proponents of the hospice movement voice their opposition to euthanasia in terms of a discourse centring upon pain, because pain is the one aspect of suffering that palliative care can often actually successfully alleviate. Even this particular success, however, may have come at a cost. One of the most common concerns expressed by staff during my fieldwork was that, once patients had ceased to be wracked by intense and interminable pain, their sensitivity to the other distressing issues which surrounded their illness and deterioration often became heightened: patients' feelings of despondency, for example, often escalated once they were in a position to be fully aware of how degrading it was to be incontinent and/or dependent upon others for their immediate bodily care. As worthwhile as the new methods of pain control have been then, the removal of one problem often leads to new problems surfacing in its place, and these latter problems may not be quite so readily resolved by palliative care.

One is thus left with the question of why the movement's concept of a 'dignified death' – articulated principally in terms of a discourse centring upon pain – has gained, and continues to have, such widespread cultural currency: a few brief ideas will have to suffice here. By suggesting that suffering can be reduced or eliminated through effective methods of pain control, hospice proponents, by sleight of hand, give the impression that suffering *is* the experience of pain *per se*. Yet, a particularly distinctive feature of physical pain, as the work of Scarry usefully highlights, is its 'unsharability'; an 'unsharability' which she suggests ensues through its resistance to language (1985: 4).[11] As she describes,

> for the person in pain, so incontestably and unnegotiably present is it that 'having pain' may come to be thought of as the most vibrant example of what it is to 'have certainty,' while for the other person it is so elusive that 'hearing about pain' may exist as the primary model of what it is 'to have doubt.' Thus pain comes unsharably into our midst as at once that which cannot be denied and that which cannot be confirmed.
>
> (Scarry 1985: 4)

As the editors of *Pain as Human Experience* similarly observe: 'Pain is an inner experience, and even those closest to the patient cannot truly observe its progress *or share in its suffering*' (Delvecchio Good *et al.* 1992: 5, emphasis added; see also Good 1992: 40; Jackson 1994: 211; D. Morris 1991: 37–8). It may well be the case, then, that the hospice movement has successfully cultivated an image of suffering as pain *per se*, because such a conception of suffering is palatable to *other people* precisely because it is 'unsharable': pain, one could argue, is by its very nature a form of sequestered suffering.

Indeed, there is much in this book to suggest that the widespread popularity behind the modern hospice movement has stemmed from the fact that it has propagated an image of dying in which others wish to believe; an image which can be sustained precisely because the suffering that patients actually experience may be hidden away in inpatient facilities, eluded and avoided in wider cultural discourses which elide suffering into pain,[12] or mystified and idealised in cultural scripts that elevate the dying to a 'heroic status' (see Seale 1998). The reality, as we have seen in this book, is often very different from that promised in the hospice formulation: dying can be a highly complex experience; one which does not, and cannot, lend itself easily to solutions, however well intended they may be (see also Nuland 1994). It may well be that, in retrospect, the pioneers of the modern hospice movement were a little too overzealous in their critique of the care of dying patients in hospitals (see Chapter 1). In highlighting the 'bodily realities of dying' this study raises the question of whether, in the end, a 'dignified death' is something we can ever realistically hope for, let alone expect.

Concluding remarks

In his now classic study *The Body Silent* (1987), the American social anthropologist Robert Murphy likened his long illness with a disease of the spinal cord to 'a kind of extended anthropological field trip', in which he 'sojourned in a social world no less strange to me at first than those of the Amazon forests' (1987: ix). As his illness progressed, he found himself drawn into ways of seeing and experiencing the world which both prompted, and enabled him, to challenge the hegemonic constructions of selfhood and sentiment in American culture. This involvement was possible precisely because the social world Murphy now found himself in was not the world of the disabled as such; it was the world he had taken for granted, until it became defamiliarised by his impairment (Thomas Couser 1997: 207).

By focusing upon the experiences of those who are dying this study, likewise, has constituted an anthropological project *par excellence*. Anthropologists who conduct fieldwork 'abroad' are often struck by 'exoticness'; that there are other ways of doing, acting and believing that are no less real, but different from, those stereotypically embedded within the anthropologist's own society. Such a phenomenon, in many cases at least, prompts the anthropologist to question the self-evident nature of his or her own (culturally inherited) assumptions and values. The 'differences' observed 'abroad', in other words, cause the anthropologist's own society to become 'visible' in new ways. This study, despite being conducted 'at home', has been very similar. It has been possible to question the self-evidentness of concepts of person and self *within* contemporary England because, in this particular cultural setting, many features that are central to the person/self only gain a visibility after they have gone: absences, like differences, create presences.

By including the experiences of patients who are very close to death, it has been possible to uncover these 'absent presences' in their starkest and most graphic forms. Many of the patients I worked with in the hospice deteriorated so fast and suddenly that they simply did not have time to make adjustments to a loss of capability or functioning before another loss (or death) occurred: presences became absent (and thus visible) in particularly marked ways. Indeed, it is extremely unlikely that this study would have developed the same depth of insights had its observations been confined solely to patients in day care (or if the focus had been upon older persons with chronic degenerative conditions or those with long-term disabilities for that matter).[13] Day care patients not only deteriorated at a significantly slower rate than their hospice counterparts, they were also able to devise a number of strategies in collaboration with staff and volunteers which enabled them to 'remake' or sustain a sense of self despite the various losses that had already ensued.[14] The absence of the autonomous aspects of patients' selves, for example, was masked and negated within day care through the formation of pseudo-surrogate family relationships which enabled exterior components of self to be emphasised instead. In fact, the tactics employed within day care were often so successful that it was not until I moved my research into the hospice, that I came to fully appreciate what exactly was being masked there. It was only by working with patients whose deterioration was so rapid that its effects could not be side-stepped or underplayed, that the central importance of bodily autonomy to selfhood gained its full visibility. The observations developed during my period of research within the hospice thus enabled me to refine (in retrospect) my analysis of the day care material, and by considering the experiences of patients in both settings in this book, it has been possible to gain a very clear and detailed understanding of what constitutes person and self in contexts such as contemporary England. It is thus with a summary of the book's theoretical contributions that I now briefly close.

This study has focused close empirical attention upon the ways in which selfhood is both lived and lost in practice in contemporary England and, in so doing, has revealed a complex and internally varied picture; one which both confirms, and challenges, the rhetorical conception of the person/self as necessarily 'rational, autonomous and unitary' (Moore 1994: 35). Conformity to 'rhetorics of individuality' (Battaglia 1995: 3) was perhaps thrown into sharpest relief in the observation that, whilst the self may vary from context to context, in all contexts (and this is crucial) *bodily autonomy* is a central (though not necessarily a sufficient criterion) for personhood. Patients experienced considerable difficulties in maintaining a sense of self once they had lost the bodily capability to 'do' and 'act' in independent ways, and, more fundamentally still, after the *physical* boundaries of their bodies had irretrievably eroded away. This latter phenomenon, in particular, indicates a concept of self which is both autonomous and interior; of a self that is 'self-contained' within the skin, isolated, alone and fenced off from other selves and from the outside world (see Chapter 5). Yet we have also seen examples which diverge from 'rhetorics of individuality'. As the interactions between carers and 'high-dependency' patients highlighted, on occasions when one person becomes the agent of another's bodily actions, the body of the latter may become merged with the body and self of the former (an observation which I also developed in my discussion of the 'making of self' through the use and incorporation of prosthetic devices). Such encounters thus point to the intersubjective and intercorporeal aspects of selfhood; to a self that is not always and necessarily mapped and experienced within an 'individuated' body, but resides within the location of (bodily) actions themselves.

In all such cases, nonetheless, it has become only too apparent that the modern 'Western' person/self cannot be understood apart from the irreducible fact of embodiment, not simply of a body of 'appearance, display and impression management', but of a body that can 'act' and can be 'self-contained'. Yet we have also seen the problems that inhere in considering the body in isolation from other factors. It is through the body that interpersonal relationships (premised upon a notion of choice and mutual autonomy) are formed and sustained, and such relationships are also a central and fundamental means by which the uniqueness of the modern 'Western' self is both realised and expressed. The self thus involves a subtle blending of interior and exterior components, an inter-weaving of bodily capabilities and relational aspects. Indeed, as the experiences of the patients described in this study have graphically highlighted, the deterioration of the body and the dissolution of the social web are often inseparable, both in interconnected ways leading to inexorable disintegration of self.

APPENDIX A

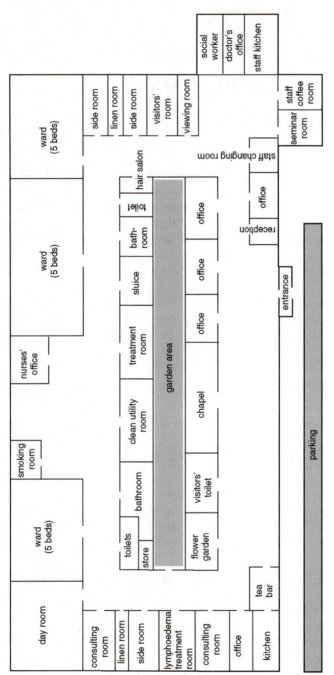

Figure The hospice

APPENDIX B

Duties of hospice in-house volunteers

The following is quoted directly from the information sheet given to all in-house volunteers who worked in the hospice during the time of the fieldwork:

The aim of having volunteers in this role is to enhance the quality and comfort of the patient's stay with us. The volunteers work alongside, and at the direction of, the trained nursing staff, their duties being complementary to those of the nursing staff.

Duties

On arrival:
Please report to the nurse-in-charge/co-ordinator as soon as you can. She will tell you what the priorities are for your session. If she is not immediately available then start on the practical tasks. The co-ordinator's name will be on the board in the nursing office.
Please check the viewing room, when not in use, for tidiness and fresh flowers.

Patient-related tasks

Spending time with patients, relatives and visitors
Offering drinks and snacks to patients and visitors where appropriate
Giving out pre-mealtime drinks, soft and alcoholic
Taking patients on outings (with staff approval)
Assisting patients with shopping as required
Writing letters for patients
Reading to patients
Sitting with patients in the day room

Assisting with any other activities e.g. jigsaw puzzles, games, sewing

Tidying bedside lockers for patients

Accompanying patients going for treatment e.g. Ray or chiropodist

Dealing with patients' flowers if necessary

Practical tasks

Stripping and making empty beds

Preparing beds and lockers for new patients

Washing small (non-soiled) laundry items if necessary

Washing bedcovers in washing machine (make sure they do *not* go to the laundry)

Returning personal laundry

Undertaking small mending tasks

Care of fridge in visitor's kitchen: check dates on foods and discard out of date or uncovered food

Washing up medicine pots

Taking full linen billies to back door and placing new bags on them

Unpacking clean linen into cupboards in bays

Emptying, washing and placing in recycling box used medicine bottles and saving any suitable for aromatherapy

Stocking up cup dispensers

Check that all patients' lockers have a name card. Spare cards are in the nurses' office

Check alcoholic drinks cupboard in Tea Bar. Inform ..., receptionist, if stocks are low

Morning volunteers: Check that cakes for afternoon tea have been taken out of the freezer and put on trolley in kitchen

Optional tasks

Hair washing and setting (a hairdresser visits on Thursdays)

Hand massage/aromatherapy (after suitable instruction from ...)

Other incidental tasks by instigation of the nurse-in-charge only

It is stressed that the volunteers assist the nurses, but in no way expect to replace nurses.

20.12.94

NOTES

1 INTRODUCTION

1 As Brody, for example, has observed, sickness can result in a 'disruption of self'; that is, 'an unpleasantly experienced break or split in a sense of personhood that ought, instead, to be felt as whole or complete' (1987: 27).

2 By using the criteria laid out by the Uniform Determination of Death Act, I take physical death to mean either the irreversible cessation of circulatory and respiratory functions, or the irreversible cessation of all functions of the entire brain including the brain stem (see Zaner 1988: 1–2).

3 Indeed, in many places in this book, it would have been impossible to avoid referring to the 'West' because this is the terminology used in much of the literature I use.

4 B. Morris, likewise, defines the person as a 'cultural category'; that is, as 'a conception articulated specifically in the cultural representations of a specific community' (1994: 11), and which impinges directly upon 'lived experience', since 'cultural representations are embedded in the practical constitution of everyday life, both social and material' (ibid.).

5 Indeed, Giddens has critiqued Goffman's idea of 'front' and 'back' regions; that is, his suggestion that persons 'enact' roles 'up front' (i.e. identities) that 'hide away' real feelings and subjective states (i.e. one's sense of self). Rather, Giddens argues for a dialectic between the two, suggesting that: 'The sustaining of ontological security could not be achieved if front regions were no more than mere façades' (1984: 125).

6 As we shall see in later chapters, patients appeared to experience a debasement of self on occasions when they became *dependent* upon family and friends for their care, and a fundamental loss of self in situations where they had become dislodged from networks of inter-personal relationships altogether.

7 See Moore (1994: 31–3) and Morris (1994: Chapter 7) for brief but incisive overviews of cross-cultural material which can be used to highlight the difficulties of assuming an elision between person and self in cultural contexts which do not share the modern 'Western' conception of individualism.

8 Since popular and academic discourses on the person/self are to some extent overlapping and mutually informing, it has sometimes been impossible to make a clear separation in this study between academic/theoretical concepts on the one hand and those used by the people I worked with on the other. Such a difficulty, needless to say, is also compounded by conducting research 'at home'.

9 It is because many of the patients I worked with experienced a debasement of personhood once their deterioration ensued that the repeated use of the term 'patient', though regrettable, has been largely unavoidable in this book. Had I chosen to use the term 'person' in place of 'patient', I would then have encountered a more fundamental problem with description and terminology in the text. Indeed, it would have been confusing to the reader (and analytically unsound) to use the term 'person' to describe someone who had entered a state of lesser or non-personhood! I do recognise, however, that the term 'patient' is not without its limitations, particularly given the nature of this study which aims to give 'a voice' to all those with whom I worked.

10 It has been necessary for me to draw upon a generalised literature examining the changing management of death and dying in the 'West', because very few writers have focused specifically on England or Britain.

11 As Pernick has observed, the appropriation of death by doctors may have originally served to enhance, at least symbolically, the status of the medical profession since, 'the power to determine death' also gave doctors 'the power to set the boundaries of life' (1988: 44).

12 In his book *Taking Rights Seriously*, the philosopher Dworkin suggests that the modern concept of rights is based upon the Kantian idea of human dignity. Rights are the entitlements of 'individuals', and thus it is inconsistent with the idea of human dignity to deprive people in any way of such recognition and treatment (1978).

13 In her discussions of the new reproductive technologies, Strathern similarly develops the idea of parents being 'customers' responding to a 'market' (1992a: 35).

14 The idea that a patient can achieve personal growth and self-enhancement through an awareness of death was also developed by the American psychiatrist Elizabeth Kübler-Ross in her book *On Death and Dying* (1969). Kübler-Ross's work provided the major impetus behind the development of the modern hospice movement in America (Abel 1986: 81).

15 However, this is a somewhat contradictory goal in the sense that inpatient facilities continue to enclave the dying processes *within* their 'bricks and mortar'.

16 The Hospice Information Service. Fact Sheet No. 4. *Architecture and Building*. London: St Christopher's Hospice Information Service.

17 *1994 Directory of Hospice Services in the UK and Republic of Ireland*. London: St Christopher's Hospice Information Service.

18 These internal market reforms passed into law through the 1990 National Health Service and Community Care Act. The reforms, in effect, caused the NHS to become divided into two halves such that there was a clear division between the 'providers' of NHS services (e.g.

NHS Trusts, NHS secondary care units and private sector units) and the 'purchasers' of such services (e.g. Health Authorities, GP fund holders and private patients) – see Holliday (1995). There have been further NHS reforms since then: at the time of writing, the government is in the process of (supposedly) abolishing the NHS internal market. In England, for example, plans are being set in motion to cease fund-holding, with the purchasing or commissioning of all health care gradually being devolved to new primary care groups (PCGs). It is expected that PCGs will develop into trusts which will not only be responsible for commissioning care, but also for providing much of it, thereby supplanting community trusts.

19 The rhetoric that home is the place where most patients would now prefer to be cared for and die will be questioned in later chapters.

20 As Saunders, the pioneer of the movement suggested: 'We moved out of the NHS in order for principles and practice to move back in' (cited in Taylor 1983: 36).

21 Walter's observation will be shown to be particularly pertinent at the end of Chapter 2, where I examine the impact that auditing procedures had upon the day care service which I studied.

22 Indeed, the use of two distinctively different languages here, the personal and emotional language of the hospice staff on the one hand, and the managerial language of rationality, systems of processes on the other, seems to be no coincidence (see James 1989).

23 A few members of the hospice staff also belonged to the Friends.

24 The visitors' kitchen was always well stocked with tea, coffee, biscuits and pre-prepared meals which were paid for with money raised by the Friends.

25 The mortuary was located in a building which was about 300 metres away from the hospice, at the main entrance of the site on which the hospice had been built.

26 The staff's rationale reflects one of the central objectives of hospice care, which is to provide patients with an environment which, as far as possible, resembles that of their own home.

27 In a survey of hospice and palliative care services in the UK in 1994–5, Eve *et al.* (1997) found that 96.7 per cent of all patients admitted to inpatient services had cancer, 1.3 per cent suffered from neurological disorders and 0.5 per cent had HIV/AIDS.

28 Staff informed me that on occasions in the past when a number of patients had died in quick succession, they did not always refill all the beds immediately. Sometimes they allowed a little time to regain their own emotional energy.

29 Such changes appear to be occurring within the hospice movement more generally. As Eve *et al.* observe in their overview of hospice and palliative care services in the UK, the national growth that has taken place in the provision of home care and day care services has been accompanied by a decline in the length of admissions to inpatient services, together with more discharges and fewer deaths per admission. Their paper focuses principally upon trends that have taken place between 1990 and 1995 (1997: 42).

30 *1994 Directory of Hospice and Palliative Care Services*. London: St Christopher's Hospice Information Service.

31 Cited from the Operational Policy of The Prince of Wales Hospice, Pontefract.

32 As Hockley and Mowatt suggest, readjustment is a better working concept to use in day care than rehabilitation, because the latter term means 'to restore to a previous condition' (1996: 13).

33 Another objective of day care was to provide a day's respite for a patient's family and other carers.

34 The day care staff have asked me to point out that the Operational Policy has been revised several times since I conducted my fieldwork.

35 It is no coincidence that an occupational therapist was appointed to this position. The rehabilitative orientation of occupational therapy is well recognised within the professional literature (see Folts *et al.* 1986; Butterfield Picard 1982).

36 According to the volunteer co-ordinator, approximately one-half of the volunteers working in day care and the hospice had lost an immediate family member or close friend due to cancer. It was fairly common for people to ask to become volunteers after a family member or friend had died in the hospice. However, the volunteer co-ordinator had a strict policy of not recruiting anyone who was recently bereaved, or who appeared to be suffering from long-term, unresolved grief. See also Hoad (1991).

37 The plethora of obstacles and difficulties I encountered during the process of setting up a fieldwork project have been documented in detail elsewhere. See Lawton (1998).

38 As I discussed earlier, audits and evaluations are now a central part of palliative care provision (Higginson 1993) and stem from recent changes in the NHS, in particular the purchaser/provider split, which has led to greater concern for quality in health care provision, and associated 'value for money' (Shaw 1993; Strong and Robinson 1990: 186).

39 All family members who were approached consented to be interviewed.

40 See also Cannon (1989) for an excellent and honest discussion of the emotional difficulties researchers encounter when working in stressful settings (Cannon worked in a hospital clinic with women who had breast cancer).

41 The staff in day care did not encounter the same problem because the service was very new and had not fully established a niche for itself.

42 Staff asked patients to state their religious persuasion on a form filled out on their admission to the hospice.

43 As a general rule, I have taken middle-class patients to be those who either worked in 'white collar' professions or had a partner in such a profession, and working-class patients to be those who worked in manual and other low-paid, low-status jobs.

2 DAY CARE: A SAFE RETREAT

1 I have borrowed the term 'alternative reality' from Hazan (1980) who used it to describe the social world constructed by participants within a day centre for elderly Jewish people in London.

2 A small number of referrals also came from district nurses and social workers. A couple of self-referrals were also made.

3 Fred's experience of social isolation also resulted from his age and position in the life course (see Chapter 5).

4 See Goffman's discussion of 'complementary stigmas', and 'stigma by association' (1963: 43).

5 See also my discussion of the 'performative' body in Chapter 3.

6 Sickness benefit was a form of financial support which could be claimed from the Department of Social Security at the time of my fieldwork if a person was pre-retirement age and too unwell to work.

7 Needless to say, this is a complicated scenario and Fiona's husband's frantic disinvestment of feelings could also be understood as a form of 'pre-mortem' bereavement.

8 See also Chapter 5 for a more detailed discussion of 'social death'.

9 Several patients told me that they were originally very anxious about going to day care because they associated this service with the hospice and thus saw their admission to day care as synonymous with a death sentence (see Chapter 1).

10 For a cross-cultural comparative perspective on disability see Ingstad and Reynolds Whyte (1995).

11 See also Littlewood 1996: 7; Murray 1993; Moore 1994: 81; Jackson 1996: 26.

12 During the planning stages of day care, the Health Commission had given its verbal support for the project. Day care's founders thus anticipated that the Health Commission would take responsibility for funding the service on a long-term basis, once the pilot had come to an end and day care had moved into its new premises (see Chapter 1).

13 Practices such as reminiscence, and the showing of family photographs, could be understood as strategies which patients usefully employed to 'imagine' and thus recreate (within day care) those relationships with family and friends that had dissipated away following the onset of their illnesses.

14 However, many patients did take advantage of a hairdressing service which was made available to them in the mornings.

15 All food and drink consumed within day care was purchased by the volunteers using money raised by the Friends. Patients could also make small donations if they chose to do so.

16 The one obvious exception to this trend was the annual trip organised by staff to a local town so that patients could do their Christmas shopping.

17 After reading the final draft of this chapter, the staff informed me that it had always been their intention to take their lead from patients. Day care, they said, was a new and innovative project, so they felt it was most appropriate to 'play things by ear'.

18 It is a well-rehearsed argument within the anthropological literature that food has a moral value and its consumption can be used as a

symbolic element in social relationships. Both Goody (1982) and Delphy (1984), for example, have observed that the consumption of food can act both as an index of equality, and as a means of reinforcing differentiation and stratification within a social group. Whilst intra-group inequality is generated and enforced through acts such as separating meal times, and the nature, content and quantity of food consumed by different members, the sharing of the same food within a communal setting, they suggest, serves to create and reflect relations of equality.

19 When patients did want to talk about their fears and anxieties about the future, it is noteworthy that they chose to do so with the staff in private rather than within the communal group setting.

20 This counsellor suggested that 'denial' and 'false hope' could hinder patients from achieving a 'good death', and could also lead to a poor outcome in bereavement for their families.

21 Kate suggested that later referrals stemmed from the fact that hospitals 'are very reluctant to let go of their patients and admit defeat until they become very unwell'.

22 This practice was not detrimental to other patients because, at the time of my fieldwork, day care did not have a substantial waiting list.

23 In fact, the majority of patients who were not re-referred had to stop coming to day care before their initial eight weeks of care had been completed, either because they became too unwell to attend, or because they had actually died.

24 The Health Commission calculated that the average cost of sending a patient through day care was approximately £700; a figure which was substantially higher than they had originally anticipated because they had not considered the possibility that patients would attend the service for longer than eight weeks. The representative went on to add that they could not justify such a high expenditure per patient when they were already having difficulties financing basic services to other patients in 'the community', such as the provision of a commode.

25 My contribution to the evaluation consisted of a simplified version of the arguments and observations developed in this chapter.

26 This is somewhat reminiscent of Evans-Pritchard's Sudanese experience as reported by Kuper (1991). Evans-Pritchard's work was not read by the colonial authorities who sponsored his research because it could not be assimilated into a predetermined quantitative framework.

3 BODY-SUBJECT TO BODY-OBJECT: HOSPICE CARE AND THE DYING PATIENT

1 Douglas' approach will be discussed further in the following chapter.

2 See Chapter 6 for a more detailed discussion.

3 See also Shilling 1991; Urla and Swedland 1995.

4 As Williams and Bendelow have observed, the conception that the 'Western' body is increasingly becoming 'plastic'; that is, an entity that can be 'moulded at will', has also been heightened by recent advances in medical science and technology. Technologies such as cosmetic

surgery, they suggest, 'greatly expand the limits of how the body may be restyled, reshaped and rebuilt' (1998: 80).

5 See, for example, Connerton (1992: 362); Lock (1993: 141–4).

6 A similar phenomenon has been pointed to by Zola (1982), a sociologist who was prompted to investigate disability partly because of his own experience of bodily impairment (Thomas Couser 1997: 211). Zola, as a result of teenage polio and a subsequent car accident, had to walk with a leg brace, back support, and a cane, though, interestingly, when he conducted fieldwork in Het Dorp – a Dutch village set up for disabled adults – he chose to use a wheelchair, so that he could experience the situation of a paraplegic first-hand. During the course of this somewhat personal fieldwork encounter, Zola experienced a notable metamorphosis of his own sense of self, his self-perception becoming that of a 'dependent', 'who could not fend for himself' (Zola 1982: 52). For other academic explorations of the lived experience of bodily impairment see, for example, Sacks (1984); Luborsky (1994); Frank (1986). An excellent overview of more auto-biographical accounts of disability can be found in Thomas Couser (1997).

7 Indeed, Murphy made the somewhat ironic comment that: 'All I can do now is read, write and talk – which is what academics call "work" ' (1987: 148).

8 A spinal cord compression occurs when a tumour in the spine grows and expands causing a breakdown of neurological functioning.

9 Penny was unable to spend more time at home because her only daughter had several young children and did not feel she had the time and resources to care for her on a full-time basis. In addition, she was ineligible for Marie Curie home care nursing support because she did not have cancer.

10 Day care patients, likewise, often brought in photographs and other memorabilia to show to other patients and staff (see Chapter 2).

11 See also Connell (1993) for a broader critique of role theory.

12 However, there are some grounds for arguing that 'industrialisation' is becoming on outdated concept. See, for example, the post-structuralist critiques provided by Battersby (1993) and Haraway (1991) that are described later on in this chapter.

13 It was common for patients to describe their cancer as a 'thing' or an 'it', implying that they saw this 'thing' or 'it' as an 'alien entity'; as an agent in its own right, which resided within them. See also Sontag (1991).

14 The same comment holds true for *The Gender of the Gift* (1988), where Strathern writes extensively about performance – exchange, transactions, production and the making of things – but not about fleshy bodies as such. In *Reproducing the Future* (1992a) and *After Nature* (1992b) Strathern does write extensively about the biological constitution of 'Western' persons, but her concern here is to explore the ways in which ideas about biology and sociality relate to one another, and not with embodiment *per se*.

15 In fact, it was only on occasions when patients made reference to aspects of their 'spoilt' bodily *appearance* that I observed any indication

of a separation and dissociation of self from body taking place. Doris, for example, frequently referred to her 'bulging' abdomen as an 'it'; an 'it' that she thereby attempted to distance from her self-image.

16 This oversight was exceptional. In no way do I wish this example to throw the competency of the hospice staff into question.

17 Glenda's poor ability to communicate, and thus to affirm the identities of the people who were significant in her life, also helps to explain why she was not seen as a social person (see Chapter 5).

18 Indeed, as I highlighted in Chapter 1, it is somewhat misleading to separate selfhood from identity (the latter term referring to the cultural meanings and social memberships conferred by others) because the two phenomena are, in practice, interlinked. As Goffman's work on stigma indicates, the body idioms people use to classify others are also used to classify the self. Hence a person with a poor bodily appearance, for example, will not only be judged by others as a 'failed' member of society, she or he will also internalise that label and thereby experience a 'spoilt' sense of self (Goffman 1963).

19 We also see this particular phenomenon (carers acting and talking for patients) ironically referred to in the title of the weekly BBC Radio 4 programme for the disabled, *Does He Take Sugar?*

20 Such a phenomenon was less evident in the interactions occurring between 'dependent' patients and professional carers (i.e. hospice staff). This may well be because the latter perform a role in which, as Gadow observes: 'The basis of the professional relation is the established disposition of one of the persons to attend to the other without receiving attention in return' (1980: 88).

21 One could argue that there is an added connection here in that an infant's body had also been carried within his or her mother's body during pregnancy, and therefore actually was a part of her body for a comparatively long period of time.

22 A similar argument has been made by Latour who argues that a simple dichotomous distinction cannot necessarily be made between 'humans' and 'non-humans' in the post-modern context. In his opinion, 'objects', like people, can have an agency in their own right (1991: 136).

23 Such a notion is also the basis of actor network theory. See, for example, Law and Hassard (1999).

24 Needless to say, there are a number of factors which continue to make it difficult for those who have severe physical impairments to achieve a fully independent lifestyle. Many shops and buildings, for example, lack viable wheelchair access. Some prosthetic devices (e.g. electronic wheelchairs and specially adapted cars) can be very expensive; hence their purchase (and the benefits that ensue from their use) is largely confined to those who are financially privileged.

25 It should be pointed out that hospice movement is fundamentally opposed to euthanasia (see Chapter 6) and the doctor did not feel that she, personally, could help a patient to die under any circumstances.

26 There are, nonetheless, some problems with the theoretical paradigms central to these studies, which I discuss at the end of the following chapter.

27 As I have described elsewhere (Lawton 1997), whilst a number of patients I spoke to in the hospice did say that witnessing another patient die could be a reassuring experience, they often added that, if they were in the same situation themselves (i.e. dying), they would prefer to be in the privacy of a side room.

28 As Lukes' study *Individualism* (1973) usefully highlights, the ideology of modern 'Western' individualism has given rise to the idea of 'natural rights', an egalitarian principle that 'asserts that respect is equally due to all persons, in virtue of their being persons, that is of some characteristic or set of characteristics they have in common' (1973: 125–6). Thus the loss of rights accorded to dying patients in the hospice could be understood as both a reflection and reinforcement of their status as 'non-persons'.

29 Staff sometimes blamed the side effects of a patient's medication in bringing about this condition. On other occasions, it was thought to result from the direct impact of the disease spread to a patient's brain.

30 Hart *et al.* (1998) have similarly argued that the ideology of the 'good death' central to the modern hospice movement is potentially highly proscriptive and can powerfully constrain the choices of dying patients.

31 However, life may, as a secondary effect, be shortened because of decreased fluid intake, movement etc. (National Council for Hospice and Specialist Palliative Care Services 1993: 8).

4 INPATIENT HOSPICE CARE: THE SEQUESTRATION OF THE UNBOUNDED BODY AND 'DIRTY DYING'

1 Taylor notes that 'caring for dying people at home appears to be a much cheaper service, at between one-quarter and one-third of the cost of an in-patient bed' (1983: 15).

2 Oedema occurs when a patient's lymphatic system becomes blocked. Lymph fluid accumulates in the limbs causing them to become very heavy and swollen.

3 Martin actually describes the women she worked with as experiencing a 'fragmentation' in which the 'self' temporarily becomes separated from the 'body'. Yet, what she appears to be highlighting here (albeit only implicitly), is the visibility that the body gains when it becomes dysfunctional (see Chapter 3); a visibility which, as Leder observes, somewhat deceptively buttresses Cartesian dualisms (1990: 86). Martin could thus be criticised for embracing the seeming appearance of a Cartesian dualism too readily in her analysis (a trap which academics such as Copp (1997) also fall into), since she does not address or fully explore the ways in which the body that appears to become 'other' at times of disruption may also affect the self. Indeed, if one carefully reads the accounts of the women Martin interviewed, experiences of a debased self during bodily trauma are only too apparent.

4 It is particularly noteworthy that children's hospices are amongst the most successful fund-raisers in the UK. Interestingly, only a small proportion of children who receive care in such settings actually have terminal cancer; the majority suffer from long-term, chronic,

debilitating conditions such as neurodegenerative disorders and muscular dystrophy (Stein *et al.* 1989). It is thus a widespread misapprehension that these particular hospices care for dying children as such (Dominica 1987); a misapprehension which, nonetheless, helps to explain their substantial success in attracting donations from the general public.

5 Carers did also point to practical factors such as the severe physical demands placed upon them by having to constantly change and launder a patient's soiled sheets. These practical concerns, nonetheless, were generally seen as secondary to the revulsion carers experienced when they were exposed to patients' bodily substances.

6 One could thus argue that – contrary to the rhetorics of community care – there are some patients at least who do not want to be cared for, or to die, at home.

7 It is at this point, needless to say, that Douglas and I part company, since Douglas does not focus her attention upon the lived, fleshy components of body 'texts' as such.

8 Such a conception of 'filth' concurs closely with Kristeva's notion of abjection (1982). For Kristeva, the abject denotes those fluid elements of the body which, when expelled, become constructed as the 'not-me'. The abject, she suggests, establishes the boundaries of the body which are also the first contours of the 'Western' subject (see Butler 1990: 133).

9 Corbin notes that public health ventures began in the seventeenth and eighteenth centuries in France (1986: 157), whereas Pasteur's discoveries did not become widespread until the 1880s (1986: 223–4). See also Cartwright (1977).

10 There are, nevertheless, some situations in which bodily unboundedness and bodily substances are not viewed negatively in 'Western' contexts. For instance, people are not generally disgusted by exchanging saliva during kissing, and having contact with other bodily fluids during consensual sexual intercourse.

11 It is interesting to note that the capacity for bodily unboundedness to disturb and disgust has also been used as a form of protest against 'the establishment': a good example being the 'dirty protests' performed by IRA H-block prisoners (see Aretxaga 1997). I was also aware of a few patients who appeared to deliberately 'unbound' their bodies (for example, by intentionally wetting themselves in bed) as a strategy for remaining in the hospice on occasions when staff were pressing for their discharge.

12 In fact neither Honeybun *et al.* (1992) nor Payne *et al.* (1996) paid explicit attention to the fact that the patients they interviewed had, in all likelihood, been exposed to the 'best' hospice deaths: it is highly likely that distressing deaths were sequestered by staff within side rooms.

5 INVISIBLE SUFFERING: THE SOCIAL DEATH

1 On 12 May 1994, Channel 4 showed a documentary, *Living with Lesley*, which was about a young woman dying of breast cancer who knew she would be leaving three young children behind. As part of the preparations for her death, Lesley made a journal for each of her children, detailing information such as their time of birth, together with other information and advice which she hoped they would want to read when they became older. In this case, Lesley appeared to be dealing with the problem of being removed from her family network by devising a means by which she could extend her 'mother identity' into the future. In contrast to Tony, Lesley had a comparatively long time (several months) to prepare for her death.

2 This is not to say that all younger patients were thought of as 'special cases'. Some young patients moved through the hospice in a fairly anonymous manner, most particularly those who had no children, were not in a long-term relationship with a partner, and had already lost their parents. Other young patients were aware of their 'terminal diagnosis' well in advance of their deaths, and had already undergone the distressing experience of being 'written off' by family and friends (see, for example, my discussion of Fiona's experiences in Chapter 2).

3 It should be pointed out, however, that this is not an implication that Strathern (1992b) actually explores in her study, because she does not recognise the possibility that kinship relationships can be lost altogether.

4 There are distinct parallels here between Giddens' conception of the 'pure relationship' as one that can be selected and deselected and Strathern's argument in *After Nature* (1992) that, in late-twentieth-century England, ideas about kinship are becoming increasingly confused with those involving consumption. Sociality, she suggests, is regarded as both a choice (implying different preferences become involved) and a human right, the implication being that people have rights, for instance, to chose children (or not, and how many), whoever they are, in the same ways as they chose different kinds of housing, furnishings and pets (1992b: Chap. 1).

5 It is noteworthy that Giddens' *The Transformation of Intimacy* (1993) does not mention the body at all, apart from one extremely brief reference to body language!

6 It is not my intention here to enter into debates about whether men and women can actually be divided in terms of their emotional responses. My concern is with actual differences in expressions of emotions (or, in this particular case, a lack of differences), which are stereotypically understood as marking gender-differentiated performances in English culture, and are therefore used to mark someone out as feminine or masculine in their behaviour.

7 Needless to say, neither Butler (1990) nor West and Zimmerman (1987) actually anticipate the possibility that gender can be lost altogether. Butler's formulation makes an assumption of body norms, whereas West and Zimmerman assume the existence of a stable social web surrounding the performer; not one that can be lost prior to death.

8 Most of the men studied by Gordon did make a recovery and, once they were able to return to sexual activities, he observed that they were able reconstruct their 'definitions of themselves as men' (1995: 254). For other examples, see Gerschick and Miller (1995); Seymour (1998); Charmaz (1995b).

9 One can see such a phenomenon occurring in its most extreme form in cases where a biologically deceased person continues to have an active (disembodied) presence in the lives of survivors. For example, in a study of elderly widows, Hallam *et al.* (1999) found that some women continued to talk to their dead spouse and to look to them for advice, thereby keeping the latter socially alive. They also point to the concept of beings such as ghosts, vampires and revenants as further examples of the biologically deceased retaining an influential social presence in the lives of others. In examples such as these it appears that certain aspects of the person/self are sustained through the continued existence of the social web that surrounded that person prior to death.

6 FINAL REFLECTIONS

1 Hinton, needless to say, is talking principally about the experiences and views of British and American people. One can also speculate that he is talking primarily about the views of those who do not come from ethnic minority backgrounds.

2 A living will (also known as an advance directive) is a document that is drawn up by a person, and witnessed by others, that lays out in some detail what should or should not be done for that person in the event of a serious illness or injury (Crowther 1993: 122). As Crowther observes, a living will often 'makes plain the person's thoughts on not wanting their life prolonged needlessly and their wish to avoid unnecessary suffering' (ibid.).

3 Significantly, in some cultural and historical contexts certain specific groups have been labelled as lesser or 'non-persons' in order to legitimate the infliction of suffering and death upon them. One obvious example is the eugenics programme which developed under Nazism. The Jews, together with other groups such as homosexuals, the congenitally weak, sick and mentally disabled were 'cast as parasites' and 'stigmatised as diseased', 'fouling the purportedly healthy German populace' (Proctor 1995: 170); hence the Nazi regime justified their mass destruction of the grounds that they were 'lives not worth living' (Harrington 1996: 191–2).

4 It hardly needs to be stated that this ideological conception meets the interests of some members of modern 'Western' societies at the expense of others. As Béteille (1983) has pointed out, the ideology of individualism serves in part to disguise and mystify the inequalities of achievement that continue to exist in contemporary 'Western' contexts. Such an argument finds support in the work of Douglas and Isherwood (1979), for example, who observe that members of the upper classes frequently hold onto their privileges (such as access to the best and most well-paid jobs) through intermarriage and the formation of closed consumption groups. Inequalities stemming from sexual dis-

crimination, racism, homophobia and ageism are also salient issues in this regard.

5 Observations such as these thus problematise the argument made by writers such as Malinowski that religion developed in societies as a way of helping 'individuals' to cope psychologically with their fear of complete annihilation (1974: 47). Such a perspective is not only grounded in a somewhat ethnocentric, 'individualistic' concept of the person, it also assumes that 'life' and 'death' are themselves self-evident concepts.

6 As I examined in Chapter 5, for example, the modern 'Western' sense of interiorised selfhood is realised and sustained through networks of interpersonal relationships and thus does have a collective aspect. Yet a crucial difference here is that relationships are often entered into as a matter of choice (Giddens' (1993) concept of the 'pure relationship'), and hence disengagement from social webs can occur before, rather than during or after death.

7 As Walker Bynum, for example, has observed, in the medieval period female mystics perceived and experienced their bodies as an open conduit linking the self to the 'sacred' and 'divine' (1989: 162–5); the body, in other words, was subordinated to higher spiritual ends (see Turner 1984: 164).

8 As I indicated in Chapter 1, the vast majority of patients who described themselves as 'religious' were from Judeo-Christian backgrounds: a phenomenon which stemmed in large part from the fact that very few patients from ethnic minority backgrounds were admitted to day care and the hospice.

9 Permission to reproduce this email message was kindly given by the author concerned.

10 Such a criticism has also been directed towards the ethics of biomedicine more generally; to the 'disembodied universalism ... so often invoked in ethical discussions' (Rothfield 1995: 169). The fact that modern 'Western' persons are, in reality, 'embodied selves' leads Diprose to suggest that, 'biomedical ethics runs the risk of being at the best ineffective and at the worst unethical' (1995: 202).

11 As Scarry observes, physical pain, unlike any other state of consciousness, has no referential content: 'It is not *of* or *for* anything' (1985: 5, original emphasis). It is because it 'takes no object that it, more than any other phenomenon, resists objectification in language' (ibid.).

12 One could go as far as to argue that, for as long as hospice proponents continue to voice their opposition to euthanasia in terms of a discourse centring primarily upon pain, the modern hospice movement constitutes little more than a red herring in contemporary debates on euthanasia.

13 This study, nonetheless, has drawn a number of parallels between the experiences of dying patients and those of the elderly and people with disabilities. Points of affinity have also been highlighted with young infants, for whom the attributes and capacities necessary for the attainment of full personhood have yet to be achieved (see Hockey and James 1993).

14 In fact, a wide range of people suffering from chronic ill health and/or a state of social isolation use tactics to preserve their selves. Reminiscence, for example, is a common (and socially sanctioned) strategy by which older persons 'imagine' and 'reinvent' relationships with people who had been significant to them at earlier stages in their lives.

BIBLIOGRAPHY

Aaronson, B. (1972) 'Behaviour and the future of time', in H. Yaker, H. Osmond and F. Cheek (eds) *The Future of Time*, New York: Anchor, pp. 405–36.

Abel, E. (1986) 'The hospice movement: institutionalising innovation', *International Journal of Health Services* 16, 1: 71–85.

Ahmedzai, S. (1993) 'The medicalization of dying', in D. Clark (ed.) *The Future For Palliative Care: Issues of Policy and Practice*, Buckingham: Open University Press, pp. 140–7.

Appadurai, A. (1986) *The Social Life of Things: Commodities in Cultural Perspective*, Cambridge: Cambridge University Press.

Ardener, S. (ed.) (1981) *Women and Space: Ground Rules and Social Maps*, London: Croom Helm.

Aretxaga, B. (1997) *Shattering Silence: Women, Nationalism and Political Subjectivity in Northern Ireland*, Chichester: Princeton University Press.

Ariès, P. (1974) *Western Attitudes Towards Death*, Baltimore: Johns Hopkins University Press.

—— (1981) *The Hour of Our Death*, London: Allen Lane.

Ariès and Bèjin (eds) (1985) *Western Sexuality: Practice and Precept in Past and Present Times*, Oxford: Basil Blackwell.

Backer, B. (1982) *Death and Dying: Individuals and Institutions*, Chichester: Wiley.

Bakhtin, M. (1968) *Rabelais and His World* (Trans. by H. Iswolsky), Cambridge Mass.: MIT Press.

Bartlett, E. and Younger, S. (1988) 'Human death and the destruction of the neocortex', in R. Zaner (ed.) *Death: Beyond Whole-Brain Criteria*, London: Kluwer Academic Publishers, pp. 199–216.

Battaglia, D. (ed.) (1995) *Rhetorics of Self-Making*, London: University of California Press.

Battersby, C. (1993) 'Her body/her boundaries: gender and the metaphysics of containment', in A. Benjamin (ed.) *Journal of Philosophy and the Visual Arts*, Special Number: The Body, pp. 31–9.

Baudrillard, J. (1981) *For a Critique of the Political Economy of the Sign*, St Louis: Telos Press.

Benson, S. (1996) 'The body, health and eating disorders', in L. Jaynes and K. Woodward (eds) *Culture, Media and Identity*, Buckingham: Open University Press.

—— (n.d.) 'Inscriptions of the self: body and identity in late capitalism', unpublished paper, Department of Social and Political Sciences, University of Cambridge.

Berger, P. and Luckmann, T. (1971) *The Social Construction of Reality: a Treatise in the Sociology of Knowledge*, London: Penguin.

Béteille, A. (1983) *The Idea of Natural Equality and Other Essays*, Oxford: Oxford University Press.

Bloch, M. (1986) *From Blessing to Violence: History and Ideology in the Circumcision Ritual of the Merina of Madagascar*, Cambridge: Cambridge University Press.

—— (1988) 'Death and the concept of the person,' in S. Cederroth, C. Corlin and J. Lindstrom (eds) *On the Meaning of Death: Essays on Mortuary Rituals and Eschatological Beliefs*, Stockholm: Almqvist & Wiksell, pp. 11–29.

Bloch, M. and Parry, J. (eds) (1982) *Death and the Regeneration of Life,* Cambridge: Cambridge University Press.

Bluebond-Langner, M. (1978) *The Private Worlds of Dying Children*, Princeton: Princeton University Press.

Bordo, S. (1993) *Unbearable Weight: Feminism, Western Culture and the Body*, London: University of California Press.

Boston, S. and Trezise, R. (1987) *Merely Mortal: Coping with Death, Dying and Bereavement*, London: Methuen.

Bourdieu, P. (1977) *Outline of a Theory of Practice*, Cambridge, Cambridge University Press.

—— (1978) 'Sport and social class', *Social Science Information* 17: 819–40.

—— (1984) *Distinction: a Social Critique of the Judgement of Taste*, Cambridge Mass.: Harvard University Press.

Brody, H. (1987) *Stories of Sickness*, London: Yale University Press.

Brotchie, J. and Hills, D. (1991) *Equal Shares in Caring: Towards Equality in Health*, London: Socialist Health Association.

Butler, J. (1990) *Gender Trouble: Feminism and the Subversion of Identity*, London: Routledge.

—— (1993) *Bodies that Matter: On the Discursive Limits of 'Sex'*, London: Routledge.

Butterfield Picard, H. (1982) 'The role of occupational therapy in hospice care', *The American Journal of Occupational Therapy* 36, 9: 597–9.

Buttimer, A. (1980) 'Social space and the planning of residential areas', in A. Buttimer and D. Seamon (eds) *The Human Experience of Space and Place*, London: Croom Helm, pp. 21–54.

Callahan, D. (1987) *Setting Limits: Medical Goals in an Aging Society*, London: Simon & Schuster.

—— (1990) 'Care of the elderly dying', in J. Walter and T. Shannon (eds) *Quality of Life: the New Medical Dilemma*, New York: Paulist Press, pp. 237–55.

Cannon, S. (1988) 'Female breast cancer: the individual experience and social organisation of its diagnosis and treatment', unpublished Ph.D. thesis, Staffordshire University.

—— (1989) 'Social research in stressful settings: difficulties for the sociologist studying the treatment of breast cancer', *Sociology of Health & Illness* 11, 1: 62–77.

Caplan, A. (1997) 'Will assisted suicide kill hospice?', in B. Jennings (ed.) *Ethics in Hospice Care: Challenges to Hospice Values in a Changing Health Environment*, London: Haworth Press, Inc., pp. 17–24.

Caplan, P. (1987) *The Cultural Construction of Sexuality*, London: Tavistock.

Cartwright, F. (1977) *A Social History of Medicine*, London: Longman.

Cassidy, S. (1994) 'The dignity of death: Frank Geden Foster Lecture', *RSA*, July: 43–55.

Charmaz, K. (1991) *Good Days, Bad Days: the Self in Chronic Illness and Time*, New Jersey: Rutgers University Press.

—— (1995a) 'The body, identity, and self: adapting to impairment', *The Sociological Quarterly* 36, 4: 657–80.

—— (1995b) 'Identity dilemmas of chronically ill men', in D. Sabo and D. F. Gordon (eds) *Men's Health and Illness: Gender, Power and the Body*, London: Sage, pp. 266–91.

Clark, D. (1993) 'Whither the hospices?', in D. Clark (ed.) *The Future for Palliative Care: Issues of Policy and Practice*, Buckingham: Open University Press, pp. 167–77.

Clark, D. and Seymour, J. (1999) *Reflections on Palliative Care*, Buckingham: Open University Press.

Classen, C., Howes, D. and Synott, A. (1994) *Aroma: the Cultural History of Smell*, London: Routledge.

Cline, S. (1995) *Lifting the Taboo: Women, Death and Dying*, London: Little, Brown and Company.

Cohen, D. and Eisdorfer, C. (1986) *The Loss of Self: a Family Resource for the Care of Alzheimer's Disease and Related Disorders*, London: W. W. Norton.

Cohen, P. (1996) 'Death duties', *Community Care* 18–24 January: 19.

Connell, R. (1993) *Gender and Power*, Cambridge: Polity Press.

—— (1995) *Masculinities*, Cambridge: Polity Press.

Connerton, P. (1992) 'Bakhtin and the representation of the body', *Journal of the Institute of Romance Studies* 1: 349–62.

Copp, G. (1997) 'Patients' and nurses' constructions of death and dying in a hospice setting', *Journal of Cancer Nursing* 1, 1: 2–13.

Corbin, A. (1986) *The Foul and the Fragrant: Odor and the French Social Imagination*, New York: Berg.

Coward, R. (1989) *The Whole Truth: the Myth of Alternative Health*, London: Faber & Faber.

Crawford, R. (1994) 'The boundaries of the self and the unhealthy other: reflections on health, culture and AIDS', *Social Science Medicine* 38, 10: 1347–65.

Crossley, N. (1995) 'Body techniques, agency and intercorporeality: on Goffman's Relations in Public', *Sociology* 29, 1: 133–49.

—— (1996) 'Body-subject/body-power: agency, inscription and control in Foucault and Merleau-Ponty', *Body & Society* 2, 2: 99–116.

Crowther, T. (1993) 'Euthanasia', in D. Clark (ed.) *The Future for Palliative Care: Issues of Policy and Practice*, Buckingham: Open University Press, pp. 111–31.

Csordas, T. (1994) (ed.) *Embodiment and Experience: the Existential Ground of Culture and Self*, Cambridge: Cambridge University Press.

Dalley, G. (1988) *Ideologies of Caring: Rethinking Community and Collectivism*, London: Macmillan Education.

Danforth, L. (1982) *The Death Rituals of Rural Greece,* Princeton, N.J.: Princeton University Press.

Davis, K. (1995) *Reshaping the Female Body: the Dilemma of Cosmetic Surgery*, London: Routledge.

Delphy, C. (1984) *Close to Home: a Material Analysis of Women's Oppression*, London: Hutchinson.

Delvecchio Good, M., Brodwin, P., Good, B. and Kleinman, A. (eds) (1992) *Pain as Human Experience: An Anthropological Perspective*, London: University of California Press.

de Raeve, L. (1994) 'Ethical issues in palliative care research', *Palliative Medicine* 8, 298–305.

Diprose, R. (1995) 'The body biomedical ethics forgets', in P. Komesaroff (ed.) *Troubled Bodies: Critical Perspectives on Postmodernism, Medical Ethics, and the Body*, London: Duke University Press, pp. 202–21.

Dominica, F. (1987) 'The role of the hospice for the dying child', *British Journal of Hospital Medicine* October: 334–43.

Douglas, M. (1970) *Natural Symbols: Explorations in Cosmology*, London: Barries & Rockliffe.

—— (1984) *Purity and Danger: an Analysis of the Concepts of Pollution and Taboo*, London: Ark.

Douglas, M. and Isherwood, B. (1979) *The World of Goods*, London: Allen Lane.

Downey, G. (1995) 'Human agency in CAD/CAM technology', in C. Gray (ed.) *The Cyborg Handbook*, New York & London: Routledge, pp. 363–70.

Downs, M. (1997) 'The emergence of the person in dementia research', *Ageing and Society* 17: 597–607.

DuBois, P. (1980) *The Hospice Way of Death*, New York: Human Sciences Press.

du Boulay, S. (1985) *Changing the Face of Death: the Story of Cicely Saunders*, London: Moral Education Press.

Dumont, L. (1985) 'A modified view of our origins: the Christian beginnings of modern individualism', in M. Carrithers, S. Collins and S. Lukes (eds) *The Category of the Person*, Cambridge: Cambridge University Press, pp. 93–122.

—— (1986) *Essays on Individualism: Modern Ideology in Anthropological Perspective*, London: University of Chicago Press.

Dunlop, R., Davies, R. and Hockley, J. (1989) 'Preferred versus actual place of death: a hospital palliative care support team experience', *Palliative Medicine* 3: 197–201.

Dworkin, R. (1978) *Taking Rights Seriously*, Cambridge Mass.: Harvard University Press.

—— (1993) *Life's Dominion: an Argument about Abortion and Euthanasia*, London: Harper Collins.

Elias, N. (1985) *The Loneliness of Dying*, Oxford: Basil Blackwell.

—— (1994) *The Civilising Process: the History of Manners and State Formation and Civilisation* (Trans. E. Jephcott), Oxford: Blackwell.

Eve, A., Smith, A. and Tebbit, P. (1997) 'Hospice and palliative care in the UK 1994–5, including a summary of trends 1990–5', *Palliative Medicine* 11: 31–43.

Ewing, K. (1990) 'The illusion of wholeness: culture, self and the experience of inconsistency', *Ethos* 18: 251–78.

Fagerhaugh, S. and Strauss, A. (1977) *Politics of Pain Management: Staff Patient Interaction*, London: Addison Wesley.

Falk, P. (1994) *The Consuming Body*, London: Sage.

—— (1995) 'Written in flesh', *Body and Society* 1, 1: 95–105.

Featherstone, M. (1993) 'The body in consumer culture', in M. Featherstone, M. Hepworth and B. Turner (eds) *The Body: Social Process and Cultural Theory*, London: Sage, pp. 170–96.

Featherstone, M. and Hepworth, M. (1993) 'The mask of ageing and the postmodern life course', in M. Featherstone, M. Hepworth and B. Turner (eds) *The Body: Social Process and Cultural Theory*, London: Sage, pp. 371–89.

Featherstone, M. and Hepworth, M. and Turner, B. (1993) (eds) *The Body: Social Process and Cultural Theory*, London: Sage.

Feifel, H. (ed.) (1959) *The Meaning of Death*, New York: McGraw-Hill.

—— (1974) 'Religious conviction and fear of death among the healthy and the terminally ill', *Journal for the Scientific Study of Religion* 13, 3: 353–60.

Fernandez, J. (1977) 'The performance of ritual metaphors', in J. Sapir and J. Crocker (eds) *The Social Use of Metaphor*, Philadelphia: University of Pennsylvania Press, pp. 100–31.

Field, D. (1996) 'Awareness of modern dying', *Mortality* 1, 3: 255–65.

Field, D. and James, N. (1993) 'Where and how people die', in D. Clark (ed.) *The Future for Palliative Care: Issues of Policy and Practice*, Buckingham: Open University Press, pp. 6–29.

Field, D. and Johnson, I. (1993) 'Volunteers in the British hospice movement', in D. Clark (ed.) *The Sociology of Death*, Oxford: Blackwell, pp. 198–217.

Fisher, R. A. and McDaid, P. (eds) (1996) *Palliative Day Care*, London: Arnold.

Folts, D., Tigges, K. and Weisman, T. (1986) 'Occupational therapy in hospice home care: a student tutorial', *The American Journal of Occupational Therapy* 40, 9: 623–8.

Fontaine, N. (1978) 'The civilizing process revisited: interview with Norbert Elias', *Theory and Society* 5, 2: 243–53.

Fontana, A. and Smith. R. (1989) 'Alzheimer's Disease victims: the "unbecoming" of self and the normalization of competence', *Sociological Perspectives* 32, 1: 35–46.

Fortes, M. (1973) 'On the concept of the person among the Tallensi', in G. Dieterlen (ed.) *La Notion de la Personne en Afrique Noire*, Paris: Editions du Centre National de le Recherche Scientifique.

Foucault, M. (1987) *The Use of Pleasure: the History of Sexuality Volume 2*, London: Penguin Books.

——— (1991) *Discipline and Punish: the Birth of the Prison*, London: Penguin Books.

——— (1993) *The Birth of the Clinic*, London: Routledge.

Frank, A. (1993) 'For a sociology of the body: an analytical review', in M. Featherstone, M. Hepworth and B. Turner (eds) *The Body: Social Process and Cultural Theory*, London: Sage, pp. 36–102.

Frank, G. (1986) 'On embodiment: a case study of congenital limb deficiency in American culture', *Culture, Medicine & Psychiatry* 10, 189–219.

Franklin, S. (1997) *Embodied Progress: a Cultural Account of Assisted Pregnancy*, London: Routledge.

Gadow, S. (1980) 'Existential advocacy: philosophical foundation of nursing', in S. Spicker and S. Gadow (eds) *Nursing: Images and Ideals*, New York: Springer Publishing Company, pp. 79–101.

——— (1989) 'Clinical subjectivity: advocacy with silent patients', *Nursing Clinics of North America* 24, 2: 535–41.

Geertz, C. (1984) ' "From the native's point of view": on the nature of anthropological understanding', in R. Shweder and R. Levine (eds) *Culture Theory: Essays on Mind, Self and Emotion*, Cambridge: Cambridge University Press, pp. 123–36.

Gell, A. (1992) *The Anthropology of Time: Cultural Constructions of Temporal Maps and Images*, Oxford: Berg.

——— (1993) *Wrapping in Images: Tattooing in Polynesia*, Oxford: Clarendon Press.

Gerhardt, U. (1990) 'Qualitative research on chronic illness: the issue and the story', *Social Science Medicine* 30, 11: 1149–59.

Gerschick, T. and Miller, A. (1995) 'Coming to terms: masculinity and physical disability', in D. Sabo and D. F. Gordon (eds) *Men's Health and Illness: Gender, Power and the Body*, London: Sage, pp. 183–204.

Giddens, A. (1979) *Central Problems in Social Theory*, Houndsmills: Macmillan.

—— (1984) *The Constitution of Society: Outline of the Theory of Structuration*, Cambridge: Polity Press.

—— (1991) *Modernity and Self-Identity*, Cambridge: Polity Press.

—— (1993) *The Transformation of Intimacy: Sexuality, Love and Eroticism in Modern Societies*, Cambridge: Polity Press.

Glaser, B. and Strauss, A. (1966) *Awareness of Dying*, Chicago: Aldine.

—— (1971) *Status Passage*, London: Routledge & Kegan Paul.

Godkin, M. (1980) 'Identity and place: clinical applications based on notions of rootedness and uprootedness', in A. Buttimer and D. Seamon (eds) *The Human Experience of Space and Place*, London: Croom Helm, pp. 73–85.

Goffman, E. (1959) *The Presentation of Self in Everyday Life*, London: Penguin Books.

—— (1962) *Relations in Public*, Harmondsworth: Penguin.

—— (1963) *Stigma: Notes on the Management of Spoilt Identity*, Englewood Cliffs, N.J.: Prentice Hall.

Golander, H. (1995) 'Rituals of temporality: the social construction of time in a nursing ward', *Journal of Aging Studies* 9, 2: 119–35.

Good, B. (1992) 'A body in pain: the making of a world of chronic pain', in M. Delvecchio Good, P. Brodwin, B. Good and A. Kleinman (eds) *Pain as Human Experience: an Anthropological Account*, London: University of California Press, pp. 29–48.

Goody, J. (1982) *Cooking, Cuisine and Class*, Cambridge: Cambridge University Press.

Gordon, D. (1990) 'Embodying illness, embodying cancer', *Culture, Medicine & Psychiatry* 14, 275–97.

Gordon, D. F. (1995) 'Testicular cancer and masculinity', in D. Sabo and D. F. Gordon (eds) *Men's Health and Illness: Gender, Power and the Body*, London: Sage, pp. 246–65.

Gorer, G. (1965) *Death, Grief and Mourning*, New York: Routledge.

Graham, H. (1983) 'Caring: a labour of love', in J. Finch and D. Groves (eds) *A Labour of Love: Women, Work and Caring*, London: RKP, pp. 13–30.

—— (1991) 'The concept of caring in feminist research: the case of domestic service', *Sociology* 25, 1: 61–78.

Green, S. (1991) 'Marking transgressions: the use of style in a women-only community in London', *Cambridge Anthropology* 15, 2: 71–87.

—— (1997) *Urban Amazons: Lesbian Feminism and Beyond in the Gender, Sexuality and Identity Battles of London*, London: Macmillan.

Griffin, J. (1991) *Dying with Dignity*, London: Office of Health Economics.

Grosz, E. (1994) *Volatile Bodies: Toward a Corporeal Feminism*, Indiana: Indiana University Press.

Gunaratnam, Y. (1997) 'Culture in not enough: a critique of multi-culturalism in palliative care', in D. Field, J. Hockey and N. Small (eds) *Death, Gender and Ethnicity*, London: Routledge, pp. 166–86.

Hallam, E., Hockey, J. and Howarth, G. (1999) *Beyond the Body: Death and Social Identity*, London: Routledge.

Haraway, D. (1991) *Simians, Cyborgs and Women: the Reinvention of Nature*, London: Free Association Books.

Harrington, A. (1996) 'Unmasking suffering's masks', *Daedalus: Journal of the American Academy of Arts and Sciences*, Social Suffering. Issued as Vol. 125, No. 1. of the Proceedings of the American Arts and Sciences, pp. 181–206.

Harris, L. (1990) 'The disadvantaged dying', *Nursing Times* 86: 26–8.

Hart, B., Sainsbury, P. and Short, S. (1998) 'Whose dying? A sociological critique of the "good death" ', *Mortality* 3, 1: 65–77.

Hazan, H. (1980) *The Limbo People: A Study of the Constitution of the Time Universe Among the Aged*, London: Routledge & Kegan Paul.

—— (1984) 'Continuity and transformation among the aged: a study in the anthropology of time', *Current Anthropology* 25, 5: 567–78.

Herskovits, E. (1995) 'Struggling over subjectivity: debates about the "self" and Alzheimer's Disease', *Medical Anthropology Quarterly* 9, 2: 146–64.

Hertz, R. (1960) *Death and the Right Hand*, London: Cohen & West.

Higginson, I. (1993) 'Clinical audit for palliative care', in I. Higginson (ed.) *Clinical Audit in Palliative Care*, Oxford: Radcliffe Medical Press, pp. 8–15.

Hilbert, R. (1984) 'The acultural dimensions of chronic pain: flawed reality construction and the problem of meaning', *Social Problems* 31, 4: 365–78.

Hill, D. and Penso, D. (1995) *Opening Doors: Improving Access to Hospice and Specialist Palliative Care Services by Members of the Black and Ethnic Minority Communities*, London: National Council for Hospice and Specialist Palliative Care Services, Occasional Paper 7.

Hinton, J. (1967) *Dying*, London: Penguin Books.

Hoad, P. (1991) 'Volunteers in the independent hospice movement', *Sociology of Health & Illness* 13, 2: 231–48.

Hobsbawm, E. and Ranger, T. (1983) *The Invention of Tradition*, Cambridge: Cambridge University Press.

Hockey, J. (1990) *Experiences of Death: an Anthropological Account*, Edinburgh: Edinburgh University Press.

Hockey, J. and James, A. (1993) *Growing Up and Growing Old: Ageing and Dependency During the Life Course*, London: Sage.

Hockley, J. and Mowatt, M. (1996) 'Rehabilitation', in R. Fisher and P. McDaid (eds) *Palliative Day Care*, London: Arnold, pp. 13–21.

Holland, A. (1984) 'Occupational therapy and day care for the terminally ill', *Occupational Therapy* Nov.: 345–8.

Holliday, I. (1995) *The NHS Transformed: a Guide to Health Reforms*, Manchester: Baseline Books.

Holmes, S. (1995) 'Ideology underpinning the issue of community care', *British Journal of Therapy and Rehabilitation* 2, 5: 246–50.

Honeybun, J., Johnson, M. and Tookman, A. (1992) 'The impact of a patient death on fellow hospice patients', *British Journal of Medical Psychology* 65: 67–72.

Hugman, R. (1994) *Power in the Caring Professions*, London: Macmillan.

Huntington, R. and Metcalf, P. (1980) *Celebrations of Death: the Anthropology of Mortuary Ritual*, Cambridge: Cambridge University Press.

Ingold, T. (1995) 'Building, dwelling, living: how animals and people make themselves at home in the world', in M. Strathern (ed.), *Shifting Contexts: Transformations in Anthropological Knowledge*, London: Routledge, pp. 57–80.

Ingstad, B. and Reynolds Whyte, S. (1995) *Disability and Culture*, California: University of California Press.

Jackson, J. (1994) 'Chronic pain and the tension between the body as subject and object', in T. Csordas (ed.) *Embodiment and Experience: the Existential Ground of Culture and Self*, Cambridge: Cambridge University Press, pp. 201–28.

Jackson, M. (1989) *Paths Towards a Clearing: Radical Empiricism and Ethnographic Enquiry*, Indiana: Indiana University Press.

—— (1996) 'Introduction: phenomenology, radical empiricism and anthropological critique', in M. Jackson (ed.) *Things as They Are: New Directions in Phenomenological Anthropology*, Indiana: Indiana University Press, pp. 1–50.

James, N. (1986) 'Care and work in nursing the dying: a participant observation study of a continuing care unit', unpublished Ph.D. thesis, Aberdeen University.

—— (1989) 'Emotional labour: skill and work in the social regulation of feelings', *Sociological Review* 37, 1: 15–42.

—— (1992) 'Care = organisation + physical labour + emotional labour', *Sociology of Health & Illness* 14, 4: 488–509.

—— (1994) 'From vision to system: the maturing of the hospice movement', in R. Lee and D. Morgan (eds) *Death Rites*, London: Routledge, pp. 102–30.

Jary, D. and Jary, J. (1995) 'The transformations of Anthony Giddens – the continuing story of structuration theory', *Theory, Culture & Society* 12, 2: 141–60.

Jenkins, D. and Price, B. (1996) 'Dementia and personhood: a focus for care?', *Journal of Advanced Nursing* 24: 84–90.

Jenkins, R. (1992) *Pierre Bourdieu*, London: Routledge.

Jennings, B. (1997) 'Individual rights and the human good in hospice', in B. Jennings (ed.) *Ethics in Hospice Care: Challenges to Hospice Values in a Changing Health Environment*, London: Haworth Press, Inc., pp. 1–8.

Jerrome, D. (1992) *Good Company: an Anthropological Study of Old People in Groups*, Edinburgh: Edinburgh University Press.

Johnson, S., Rogers, C., Biswas, B. and Ahmedzai, S. (1990) 'What do hospices do? A survey of hospices in the United Kingdom and the Republic of Ireland', *British Medical Journal* 300: 791–3.

Kastenbaum, R. and Aisenberg, R. (1974) *The Psychology of Death*, London: Duckworth.

Kearl, M. (1989) *Endings: a Sociology of Death and Dying*, Oxford: Oxford University Press.

Kelly, M. and Field, D. (1996) 'Medical sociology, chronic illness and the body', *Sociology of Health & Illness* 18, 2: 241–57.

Kleinman, A. (1988) *The Illness Narratives: Suffering, Healing and the Human Condition*, New York: Basic Books.

Kleinman, A. and Kleinman, J. (1996) 'The appeal of experience; the dismay of images: cultural appropriations in our times', *Daedalus: Journal of the American Arts and Social Sciences*, Social Suffering. Issued as Vol. 125, No. 1. Proceedings of the American Academy of Arts and Sciences, pp. 1–23.

Kleinman, A., Das, V. and Lock, M. (1996) 'Introduction', *Daedalus: Journal of the American Arts and Social Sciences*, Social Suffering. Issued as Vol. 125, No. 1. Proceedings of the American Academy of Arts and Sciences, pp. xi–xx.

Kristeva, J. (1982) *Powers of Horror: an Essay on Abjection* (Trans. L. Roudiez), New York: Columbia University Press.

Kritjanson, L., Hanson, E. and Belneaves, L. (1994) 'Research in palliative care: ethical issues', *Journal of Palliative Care* 10, 3: 10–15.

Kübler-Ross, E. (1969) *On Death and Dying*, London: Tavistock.

Kuper, A. (1991) *Anthropology and Anthropologists: the Modern British School*, London: Routledge.

La Fontaine, J. (1985) 'Person and individual: some anthropological reflections', in M. Carrithers, S. Collins and S. Lukes (eds) *The Category of the Person*, Cambridge: Cambridge University Press, pp. 123–40.

—— (1990) *Child Sexual Abuse*, Cambridge: Polity Press.

—— (1996) 'Organised and ritual abuse', *Medicine, Science and the Law* 36, 2: 109–17.

Lakoff, G. and Johnson, M. (1980) *Metaphors We Live By*, London: University of Chicago Press.

Lamb, D. (1990) *Organ Transplants and Ethics*, London: Routledge.

Langer, L. (1996) 'The alarmed vision: social suffering and the holocaust atrocity', *Daedalus: Journal of the American Arts and Social Sciences*. Social Suffering. Issued as Vol. 125, No. 1. Proceedings of the American Academy of Arts and Sciences, pp. 47–65.

Langer, M. (1989) *Merleau-Ponty's Phenomenology of Perception: a Guide and Commentary*, Basingstoke: Macmillan.

Laqueur, T. (1992) *Making Sex: Body and Gender from the Greeks to Freud*, London: Harvard University Press.

Lasch, C. (1977) *Haven in a Heartless World*, New York: Basic Books.

Latour, B. (1991) *We Have Never Been Modern*, London: Harvester Wheatsheaf.

Law, J. and Hassard, J. (eds) (1999) *Actor Network Theory and After*, Oxford: Blackwell.

Lawler, J. (1991) *Behind the Screens: Nursing Somology and the Body*, London: Churchill Livingstone.

Lawton, J. (1997) 'A room with a view: dying and dignity in the hospice setting', *Nursing Times*, 20 August: 53–4.

—— (1998) 'The disintegration of self: a study of patients in a day care service and a hospice in England', unpublished Ph.D. thesis, University of Cambridge.

Leder, D. (1990) *The Absent Body*, Chicago: University of Chicago Press.

Lee, R. and Morgan, D. (eds) (1994) *Death Rites: Law and Ethics at the End of Life*, London: Routledge.

Lewis, J. (ed.) (1986) *Labour and Love: Women's Experiences of Home and Family, 1850–1940*, Oxford: Basil Blackwell.

Lifton, R. (1967) *Death in Life: Survivors of Hiroshima*, New York: Random House.

Littlewood, R. (1996) *Reason and Necessity in the Specification of the Multiple Self*, Royal Anthropological Institute, Occasional Paper 43.

Lloyd, G. (1993) *Being in Time: Selves and Narrators in Philosophy and Literature*, London: Routledge.

Lock, M. (1993) 'Cultivating the body: anthropology and epistemologies of bodily practice and knowledge', *Annual Review of Anthropology* 22: 133–55.

—— (1996) 'Displacing suffering: the reconstruction of death in North America and Japan', *Daedalus: Journal of the American Arts and Social Sciences*. Social Suffering. Issued as Vol. 125, No. 1. Proceedings of the American Academy of Arts and Sciences, pp. 207–44.

Lofland, L. (1978) *The Craft of Dying: the Modern Face of Death*, London: Sage.

Luborsky, M. (1994) 'The cultural adversity of physical disability: erosion of full adult personhood', *Journal of Aging Studies* 8, 3: 239–53.

Luckmann, T. (1967) *The Invisible Religion: the Problem of Religion in Modern Society*, London: Macmillan.

Lukes, S. (1973) *Individualism*, Oxford: Basil Blackwell.

—— (1985) 'Conclusion', in M. Carrithers, S. Collins and S. Lukes (eds) *The Category of the Person*, Cambridge: Cambridge University Press, pp. 282–301.

Lunt, B. (1985) 'Terminal cancer care services: recent changes in regional inequalities in Great Britain', *Social Science Medicine* 20, 7: 753–9.

Lutz, C. (1988) *Unnatural Emotions: Everyday Sentiments on a Micronesian Atoll and their Challenge to Western Theory*, London: University of Chicago Press.

Lutz, C. and White, G. (1986) 'The anthropology of emotions', *Annual Review of Anthropology* 15: 405–36.

McCormick, R. (1990) 'To save or let die', in J. Walter and T. Shannon (eds) *Quality of Life: the New Medical Dilemma*, New York: Paulist Press.

McCourt Perring, C. (1994) 'Community care as de-institutionalization: continuity and change in the transition from hospital to community-based care', in S. Wright (ed.) *Anthropology of Organisations*, London: Routledge, pp. 168–80.

Macfarlane, A. (1978) *The Origins of English Individualism*, Oxford: Basil Blackwell.

McNamara, B., Waddel, D. and Colvin, M. (1994) 'The institutionalisation of the good death', *Social Science Medicine* 39, 11: 1501–8.

Malinowski, B. (1974) *Magic, Science and Religion*, London: Souvenir Press.

Martin, E. (1989) *The Woman in the Body: a Cultural Analysis of Reproduction*, Buckingham: Open University Press.

Mascia-Lees, P. and Sharpe, P. (eds) (1992) *Tattoo, Mutilation, and Adornment: the Denaturalization of the Body in Culture and Text*, Albany: State University of New York Press.

Mauss, M. (1985) 'A category of the human mind: the notion of the person; the notion of the self', in M. Carrithers, S. Collins and S. Lukes (eds) *The Category of the Person*, Cambridge: Cambridge University Press, pp. 1–25.

—— (1990) *The Gift: the Form and Reason for Exchange in Archaic Societies*, London: Routledge.

—— (1992) [1934] 'Techniques of the body', in J. Crary and S. Kwinter (eds) *Incorporations*, New York: Zone.

Mead, G. H. (1934) *Mind, Self and Society: From the Standpoint of a Social Behaviourist*, Chicago: Chicago University Press.

Medick, H. and Sabean, D. (1984) *Interest and Emotion: Essays on the Study of Family and Kinship*, Cambridge: Cambridge University Press.

Meigs, A. (1984) *Food, Sex, and Pollution: a New Guinea Religion*, New Jersey: Rutgers University Press.

Mellor, P. (1993) 'Death in high modernity: the contemporary presence and absence of death', in D. Clark (ed.) *The Sociology of Death*, Oxford: Blackwell, pp. 11–30.

Merleau-Ponty, M. (1962) *Phenomenology of Perception*, London: Routledge & Kegan Paul.

Meyer, R. (1991) 'Rock Hudson's body', in D. Fuss (ed.) *Inside/Out: Lesbian Theories, Gay Theories*, London: Routledge, pp. 259–88.

Miller, D. (1988) 'Appropriating the state on the council estate', *Man* 23, 2: 353–72.

—— (1991) *Material Culture and Mass Consumption*, Oxford: Basil Blackwell.

Mitteness, L. and Barker, C. (1995) 'Stigmatizing a "normal" condition: urinary incontinence in later life', *Medical Anthropology Quarterly* 9, 2: 188–210.

Moller, D. (1996) *Confronting Death: Values, Institutions and Human Mortality*, Oxford: Oxford University Press.

Moore, H. (1994) *A Passion for Difference: Essays in Anthropology and Gender*, Cambridge: Polity Press.

Morris, B. (1991) *Western Conceptions of the Individual*, Oxford: Berg.

—— (1994) *The Anthropology of the Self: the Individual in Cultural Perspective*, London: Pluto Press.

Morris, D. (1991) *The Culture of Pain*, California: University of California Press.

Mulkay, M. (1993) 'Social death in Britain', in D. Clark (ed.) *The Sociology of Death*, Oxford: Blackwell, pp. 31–49.

Munley, A. (1983) *The Hospice Alternative*, New York: Basic Books.

Munn, N. (1992) 'The cultural anthropology of time: a critical essay', *Annual Review of Anthropology* 21: 93–123.

Murphy, M. (1993) 'Confusion', in C. Saunders and N. Sykes (eds) *Terminal Malignant Disease*, London: Hodder & Stoughton, pp. 131–8.

Murphy, R. (1987) *The Body Silent*, London: Phoenix House.

Murray, D. (1993) 'What is the Western concept of self? On forgetting David Hume', *Ethos* 21, 1: 3–23.

National Council for Hospice and Specialist Palliative Care Services (1993) *Key Ethical Issues in Palliative Care: Evidence to House of Lords Select Committee on Medical Ethics*, Occasional Paper 3.

Neale, B. (1993) 'Informal care and community care', in D. Clark (ed.) *The Future for Palliative Care: Issues of Policy and Practice*, Buckingham: Open University Press, pp. 52–67.

Nuland, S. (1994) *How We Die*, London: Chatto & Windus.

O'Brien, T. (1993) 'Pain', in C. Saunders and N. Sykes (eds) *Terminal Malignant Disease*, London: Hodder & Stoughton, pp. 33–62.

Orona, C. (1990) 'Temporality and identity loss due to Alzheimer's disease', *Social Science Medicine* 30, 11: 1247–56.

Ortner, S. (1984) 'Theory in anthropology since the sixties', *Comparative Study of Society and History* 126–66.

Owens, P. (1995) 'Palliative care', in P. Owens, J. Carrier and J. Horder (eds) *Interprofessional Issues in Community and Primary Health Care*, London: Macmillan, pp. 165–83.

Parker, G. (1990) 'Spouse carers: whose quality of life?', in S. Baldwin, C. Godfrey and C. Propper (eds) *Quality of Life: Perspectives and Policies*, London: Routledge, pp. 120–30.

Parry, J. (1982) 'Sacrificial death and the necrophagous ascetic', in M. Bloch and J. Parry (eds) *Death and the Regeneration of Life*, Cambridge: Cambridge University Press, pp. 74–110.

—— (1994) *Death in Banaras*, Cambridge: Cambridge University Press.

Payne, S., Hillier, R., Langley-Evans, A. and Roberts, T. (1996) 'Impact of witnessing death on hospice patients', *Social Science Medicine* 43, 12: 1785–94.

Pernick, R. (1988) 'Back from the grave', in R. Zaner (ed.) *Death: Beyond Whole-Brain Criteria*, London: Kluwer Academic Publishers, pp. 17–74.

Pines, D. (1993) '*A Woman's Unconscious Use of Her Body: a Psychoanalytical Perspective*, London: Virago Press.

Proctor, R. (1995) 'The destruction of "lives not worth living" ', in J. Terry and J. Urla (eds) *Deviant Bodies: Critical Perspectives on Difference in Science and Popular Culture*, Indiana: Indiana University Press, pp. 170–96.

Randall, F. and Downie, R. (1996) *Palliative Care Ethics: a Good Companion*, Oxford: Oxford University Press.

Richardson, R. (1989) *Death, Dissection and the Destitute*, Harmondsworth: Penguin Books.

Robillard, A. (1996) 'Anger in-the-social-order', *Body & Society* 2, 1: 17–30.

Roper, M. (1994) 'Gender and organizational change', in S. Wright (ed.) *Anthropology of Organizations*, London: Routledge, pp. 87–94.

Rose, N. (1990) *Governing the Soul: the Shaping of the Private Self*, London: Routledge.

—— (1996) *Inventing Our Selves: Psychology, Power and Personhood*, Cambridge: Cambridge University Press.

Rothfield, P. (1995) 'Bodies and subjects: medical ethics and feminism', in P. Komesaroff (ed.) *Troubled Bodies: Critical Perspectives on Postmodernism, Medical Ethics, and the Body*, Duke: Duke University Press, pp. 168–201.

Rowles, G. (1980) 'Toward a geography of growing old', in A. Buttimer and D. Seamon (eds) *The Human Experience of Space and Place*, London: Croom Helm, pp. 55–72.

Sacks, O. (1984) *A Leg to Stand On*, London: Duckworth.

Said, E. (1991) *Orientalism: Western Conceptions of the Orient*, Harmondsworth: Penguin.

Sartre, J. (1956) *Being and Nothingness: a Phenomenological Essay on Nothingness* (Trans. H. Barnes), New York: Pocket Books.

Saunders, C. (1965) 'Watch with me', *Nursing Times* Nov. 2 (reprint obtained from St Christopher's Hospice Information Service, London).

—— (1986) 'The last refuge', *Nursing Times* Oct. 2: 28–30.

—— (1988) 'Spiritual pain', *Hospital Chaplain* March (reprint obtained from St Christopher's Hospice Information Service, London).

—— (1992) 'Voluntary euthanasia', *Palliative Medicine* 6: 1–5.

—— (1993a) 'Introduction – "history and challenge" ', in C. Saunders and N. Sykes (eds) *Terminal Malignant Disease*, London: Hodder & Stoughton, pp. 1–14.

—— (1993b) 'Some challenges that face us', *Palliative Medicine* 7 (supplement 1): 77–83.

Scarry, E. (1985) *The Body in Pain: the Making and Unmaking of the World*, New York: Oxford University Press.

Schutz, A. (1967) 'On multiple realities', in M. Natanson (ed.) *Alfred Schutz Collected Papers 1: the Problem of Social Reality*, The Hague: Martinus Nijhoff.

Scott, J. (1994) 'More money for palliative care? The economics of denial', *Journal of Palliative Care* 10, 3: 35–8.

Seale, C. (1989) 'What happens in hospices: a review of research evidence', *Social Science Medicine* 28, 6: 551–9.

—— (1990) 'Demographic change and the care of the dying, 1969–1987', in D. Dickenson and M. Johnson (eds) *Death, Dying and Bereavement*, London: Sage, pp. 45–54.

—— (1998) *Constructing Death: the Sociology of Dying and Bereavement*, Cambridge: Cambridge University Press.

Seale, C. and Addington-Hall, J. (1995) 'Euthanasia: the role of good care', *Social Science and Medicine* 40, 5: 581–7.

Seymour, W. (1998) *Remaking the Body: Rehabilitation and Change*, London: Routledge.

Sharma, U. (1992) *Complimentary Medicine Today: Practitioners and Patients*, London: Routledge.

Shaw, C. (1993) 'Introduction to audit in palliative care', in I. Higginson (ed.) *Clinical Audit in Palliative Care*, Oxford: Radcliffe Medical Press, pp. 1–7.

Shilling, C. (1991) 'Educating the body: physical capital and the production of social inequalities', *Sociology* 25, 4: 653–72.

—— (1993) *The Body and Social Theory*, London: Sage.

Shilling, C. and Mellor, P. (1996) 'Embodiment, structuration theory and modernity: mind/body dualism and the repression of sensuality', *Body & Society* 2, 4 : 1–15.

Shore, B. (1982) *Sala'ilua: a Samoan Mystery*, New York: Columbia University Press.

Skeggs, B. (1997) *Formations of Class and Gender*, London: Sage.

Skinner Cook, A. and Oltjenburns, K. (1989) *Dying and Grieving: Lifespan and Family Perspectives*, London: Holt, Rinehart and Winston Inc.

Smaje, C. and Field, D. (1997) 'Absent minorities? Ethnicity and the use of palliative care services', in D. Field, J. Hockey and N. Small (eds) *Death, Gender and Ethnicity*, London: Routledge, pp. 142–65.

Smith, A. (1989) *Helping the Dying*, London: St Christopher's Hospice Information Service.

Sontag, S. (1991) *Illness as Metaphor – Aids and its Metaphors*, London: Penguin Books.

Standing Medical Advisory Committee and Standing Nursing and Midwifery Advisory Committee (1993) *The Principles and Provision of Palliative Care*, Joint Report of the Standing Medical Advisory Committee and Standing Nursing and Midwifery Committee 1992, London: HMSO.

Stein, A., Forrest, G., Woolley, H. and Baum, J. (1989) 'Life threatening illness and hospice care', *Archives of Disease in Childhood* 64: 697–702.

Stone, S. (1995) 'Split subjects, not atoms; or how I fell in love with my prosthesis', in C. Gray (ed.) *The Cyborg Handbook*, New York & London: Routledge, pp. 393–406.

Strathern, M. (ed.) (1987) *Dealing with Inequality: Analysing Gender Relations in Melanesia and Beyond*, Cambridge: Cambridge University Press.

—— (1988) *The Gender of the Gift: Problems with Women and Problems with Society in Melanesia*, London: University of California Press.

—— (1992a) *Reproducing the Future: Anthropology, Kinship and the New Reproductive Technologies*, Manchester: Manchester University Press.

—— (1992b) *After Nature: English Kinship in the Late Twentieth Century*, Cambridge: Cambridge University Press.

Strong, P. and Robinson. J. (1990) *The NHS – Under New Management*, Buckingham: Open University Press.

Sudnow, D. (1967) *Passing On: the Social Organisation of Dying*, Englewood Cliffs, N.J.: Prentice Hall.

Süskind, P. (1987) *Perfume: the Story of a Murderer*, London: Penguin Books.

Taylor, C. (1985) 'The person', in M. Carrithers, S. Collins and S. Lukes (eds) *The Category of the Person*, Cambridge: Cambridge University Press, pp. 257–81.

—— (1989) *Sources of Self: the Making of Modern Identity*, Cambridge: Cambridge University Press.

Taylor, C. C. (n.d.) 'Fluids and fractals in Central Africa', unpublished paper, Anthropology Department, University of Alabama.

Taylor, H. (1983) *The Hospice Movement in Britain: its Role and its Future*, London: Centre for Policy an Ageing.

Thomas, C. (1993) 'De-constructing concepts of care', *Sociology* 27, 4: 649–69.

Thomas Couser, G. (1997) *Recovering Bodies: Illness, Disability and Life Writing*, Wisconsin: University of Wisconsin Press.

Thorpe, G. (1993) 'Enabling more dying people to remain at home', *British Medical Journal* 307: 915–18.

Toombs, S. (1995) 'The lived experience of disability', *Human Studies* 18: 9–23.

Torrens, P. (1986) 'U.S. hospice between two worlds', *Journal of Palliative Care* 2: 6–8.

Townsend, J., Frank, A., Fermont, D., Dyer, S. and Karran, O. (1990) 'Terminal cancer care and patients preference for death: a prospective study', *British Medical Journal* 301, 415–17.

Treichler, P. (1990) 'Feminism, medicine and the meaning of childbirth', in M. Jacobus, E. Fox Keller and S. Shuttleworth (eds) *Body/Politics: Women and the Discourses of Science*, London: Routledge, 113–38.

Turner, B. (1984) *The Body and Society*, Oxford: Basil Blackwell.

BIBLIOGRAPHY

—— (1992) *Regulating Bodies: Essays in Medical Sociology*, London: Routledge.

Turner, V. (1967) *The Forest of Symbols: Aspects of Ndembu Ritual*, Ithaca: Cornell University Press.

Twycross, R. (1986) *A Time to Die*, London: Christian Medical Fellowship.

—— (1992) *The Dying Patient*, London: Christian Fellowship.

Ungerson, C. (1987) *Policy is Personal*, London: Tavistock.

Urla, J. and Swedland, A. (1995) 'The anthropometry of Barbie: unsettling ideals of the feminine body in popular culture', in J. Terry and J. Urla (eds) *Deviant Bodies*, Bloomington: Indiana University Press, pp. 277–313.

Van Gennep, A. (1972) *The Rites of Passage*, Chicago: University of Chicago Press.

Vialles, N. (1994) *Animal to Edible*, Cambridge: Cambridge University Press.

Walker Bynum, C. (1989) 'The female body and religious practices in the later Middle Ages', in M. Feher (ed.) *Fragments for a History of the Human Body. Part 1*, New York: Zone, pp. 160–219.

Walter, J. and Shannon, T. (eds) (1990) *Quality of Life: the New Medical Dilemma*, New York: Paulist Press.

Walter, T. (1993) 'Sociologists never die: British sociology and death', in D. Clark (ed.) *The Sociology of Death*, Buckingham: Open University Press, pp. 264–95.

—— (1994) *The Revival of Death*, London: Routledge.

Watson, J. (1982) 'Of flesh and bones: the management of death pollution in Cantonese society', in M. Bloch and J. Parry (eds) *Death and the Regeneration of Life*, Cambridge: Cambridge University Press, 155–86.

Webb, C. (1985) *Sexuality, Nursing and Health*, Chichester: Wiley.

Weeks, J. (1986) *Sexuality*, London: Routledge.

Weisman, A. (1979) *Coping with Cancer*, London: McGraw-Hill.

Weiss, G. (1999) *Body Images: Embodiment as Intercorporeality*, London: Routledge.

West, C. and Zimmerman, D. (1987) 'Doing gender', *Gender & Society* 1, 2: 125–51.

White, P. (1988) 'Should the law define death?', in R. Zaner (ed.) *Death: Beyond Whole-Brain Criteria*, London: Kluwer Academic Publishers, pp. 101–9.

Wilkes, E. (1993) 'Introduction', in D. Clark (ed.) *The Future for Palliative Care: Issues of Policy and Practice*, Buckingham: Open University Press, pp. 1–5.

Williams, S. (1995) 'Theorising class, health and lifestyles: can Bourdieu help us?', *Sociology of Health & Illness* 17, 5: 577–604.

—— (1996) 'The vicissitudes of embodiment across the chronic illness trajectory', *Body & Society* 2, 2: 22–47.

Williams, S. and Bendelow, G. (1998) *The Lived Body: Sociological Themes, Embodied Issues*, London: Routledge.

Woodburn, J. (1982) 'Social dimensions of death in four African hunting and gathering societies', in M. Bloch and J. Parry (eds) *Death and the Regeneration of Life*, Cambridge: Cambridge University Press, pp. 187–210.

Woodhall, C. (1986) 'Care of the dying: a family concern', *Nursing Times* Oct. 22: 31–3.

Wright, S. (1994) 'Culture in anthropology and organisational studies', in S. Wright (ed.) *The Anthropology of Organisations*, London: Routledge, pp. 1–31.

Zaner, R. (ed.) (1988) *Death: Beyond Whole-Brain Criteria*, London: Kluwer Academic Publishers.

Zaretsky, E. (1976) *Capitalism, the Family and Personal Life*, London: Pluto Press.

Zola, I. (1982) *Missing Pieces: Chronicle of Living with a Disability*, Philadelphia: Temple University Press.

Zussman, R. (1992) *Intensive Care: Medical Ethics and the Medical Profession*, London: The University of Chicago Press.

NAME INDEX

Aaronson, B. 100
Abel, E. 12, 13, 14, 19
Addington-Hall, J. 179
Ahmedzai, S. 18, 19
Aisenberg, R. 15, 143
Anzieu, D. 139
Appadurai, A. 92
Ardener, S. 54–5, 97, 100–1
Aretxaga, B. 200
Ariès, P.: (1974) 119, 143; (1981)
    8–10, 114, 119, 145; and Bèjin
    (1985) 168; Elias on 11

Backer, B. 10, 171, 173
Bakhtin, M. 138
Barker, C. 142
Bartlett, E. 115
Battaglia, D. 7, 184
Battersby, C. 110–11, 197
Baudrillard, J. 92
Bendelow, G. 162, 196
Benson, S. 83–4, 139
Berger, P. 161
Béteille, A. 202
Bloch, M. 7, 173–4
Bluebond-Langner, M. 49
Bordo, S. 83, 139
Boston, S. 47
Bourdieu, P. 83, 137, 169–70
Brody, H. 191
Brotchie, J. 23, 60, 165
Butler, J. 53, 167, 168, 200, 201
Butterfield Picard, H. 194
Buttimer, A. 54–5

Callahan, D. 172

Cannon, S. 168, 194
Caplan, A. 178, 180
Caplan, P. 168
Cartwright, F. 200
Cassidy, S. 179
Charmaz, K. 46, 87, 202
Clark, D. 18, 19, 133, 180
Classen, C. 136
Cline, S. 9
Cohen, D. 116
Cohen, P. 133
Connell, R. 167, 197
Connerton, P. 197
Copp, G. 199
Corbin, A. 136, 141, 200
Coward, R. 14, 83
Crawford, R. 83, 138, 139
Crossley, N. 58, 83, 90, 101, 162
Crowther, T. 202
Csordas, T. 82, 83, 85

Dalley, G. 61
Danforth, L. 173, 174
Davis, K. 45
de Raeve, L. 30
Delphy, C. 196
Delvecchio Good, M. 182
Diprose, R. 85, 203
Dominica, F. 200
Douglas, M.: (1970) 82; (1984) 82,
    136, 137, 141, 174; and
    Isherwood (1979) 92, 202
Downey, G. 110
Downie, R. 30
Downs, M. 115
du Boulay, S. 12

DuBois, P. 12
Dumont, L. 4, 6, 173
Dunlop, R. 122
Dworkin, R. 132, 192

Eisdorfer, C. 116
Elias, N. 6, 11, 117, 138, 141, 145
Eve, A. 34, 123, 128, 193

Fagerhaugh, S. 15, 119, 120, 132
Falk, P. 1, 7, 83, 101
Featherstone, M. 1, 7, 83, 84, 175
Feifel, H. 175
Fernandez, J. 94
Field, D.: (1996) 93, 133; and James (1993) 9, 13; and Johnson (1993) 17; Kelly and (1996) 84; Smaje and (1997) 34
Fisher, R.A. 23, 24
Folts, D. 194
Fontaine, N. 138
Fontana, A. 115
Fortes, M. 4
Foucault, M.: (1987) 6; (1991) 101, 118, 138; (1993) 9, 60; influence 82
Frank, A. 83
Frank, G. 197
Franklin, S. 6

Gadow, S. 118, 121, 198
Geertz, C. 109
Gell, A. 47, 67, 139
Gerhardt, U. 172
Gerschick, T. 202
Giddens, A.: (1979) 102; (1984) 58, 59, 102, 191; (1991) 1, 5, 8, 13, 38, 83, 161–2; (1993) 8, 38, 161–2, 201, 203; on autonomy 165; on pure relationship 164–5, 201
Glaser, B. 10, 113, 153
Godkin, M. 54
Goffman, E.: (1959) 5, 38, 53, 54, 83, 162; (1962) 162; (1963) 38, 45, 163, 195, 198; Crossley on 90; Giddens on 191; influence 162–3
Golander, H. 47–8, 66
Good, B. 182
Goody, J. 196
Gordon, D. 49, 81
Gordon, D.F. 168

Gorer, G. 10, 114, 143
Graham, H. 61, 65
Green, S. 101
Griffin, J. 18
Grosz, E. 108, 131, 142–3
Gunaratnam, Y. 34

Hallam, E. 202
Haraway, D. 110, 197, 111
Harrington, A. 202
Harris, L. 133
Hart, B. 199
Hassard, J. 198
Hawking, S. 112
Hazan, H. 57, 67, 100, 154, 195
Hepworth, M. 84
Herskovits, E. 115
Hertz, R. 82, 173
Higginson, I. 194
Hill, D. 34
Hills, D. 23, 60, 165
Hinton, J. 171, 175, 202
Hoad, P. 194
Hobsbawm, E. 11
Hockey, J.: (1990) 9, 10, 15, 133, 145, 159–60; and James (1993) 52, 60, 65, 142, 203
Hockley, J. 24, 194
Holliday, I. 193
Holmes, S. 122
Honeybun, J. 15, 118, 146, 200
Hugman, R. 19, 61, 73
Huntington, R. 173

Ingold, T. 55
Ingstad, B. 195
Isherwood, B. 92, 202

Jackie (Macmillan nurse) 41, 47
Jackson, J. 46, 182
Jackson, M. 5, 82, 87, 94, 195
James, A. 52, 60, 65, 142, 203
James, N.: (1986) 19, 180; (1989) 193; (1992) 61–2; (1994) 12, 17, 19, 180; Field and (1993) 9, 13
Jary, D. 162
Jary, J. 162
Jenkins, D. 115
Jenkins, R. 170
Jennings, B. 179

Jerrome, D. 56
Johnson, I. 17
Johnson, M. 94
Johnson, S. 19

Kastenbaum, R. 15, 143
Kearl, M. 9, 13, 154, 170
Kelly, M. 84
Kleinman, A. 74–5, 175
Kleinman, J. 74–5
Kristeva, J. 200
Kritjanson, L. 30
Kübler-Ross, E. 47, 49, 79, 175, 192
Kuper, A. 196

La Fontaine, J. 4, 6, 61, 64–5, 109, 173
Lakoff, G. 94
Lamb, D. 115
Langer, L. 131, 155–6
Langer, M. 97
Laqueur, T. 168
Lasch, C. 161
Latour, B. 198
Law, J. 198
Lawler, J. 60, 117, 118
Lawton, J. 194, 199
Leder, D. 84–6, 94, 102, 108, 199
Lee, R. 132
Lewis, J. 61
Lifton, R. 131
Littlewood, R. 195
Lloyd, G. 5
Lock, M. 82, 197
Lofland, L. 172
Luborsky, M. 197
Luckmann, T. 160–1
Lukes, S. 6, 199
Lunt, B. 12, 17, 18, 23, 122
Lutz, C. 61, 63

McCormick, R. 156
McCourt Perring, C. 54
McDaid, P. 23, 24
Macfarlane, A. 6, 109
McNamara, B. 119
Malinowski, B., 203
Martin, E. 131, 199
Mascia-Lees, P. 83
Mauss, M. 4, 6, 66, 137
Mead, G.H. 5

Medick, H. 63
Meigs, A. 137, 140, 141
Mellor, P. 102, 123, 143, 162
Merleau-Ponty, M. 87, 90, 96, 103
Metcalf, P. 173
Meyer, R. 144
Miller, A. 202
Miller, D. 15, 92
Mitteness, L. 142
Moller, D. 12, 16, 19, 143, 145
Moore, H. 3, 7, 41, 58, 110, 184, 191, 195
Morgan, D. 132
Morris, B. 5, 6, 7, 191
Morris, D. 134, 182
Mowatt, M. 24, 194
Mulkay, M. 14, 51
Munley, A. 12
Munn, N. 67
Murphy, M. 14
Murphy, R. 85–6, 182, 197
Murray, D. 195

National Council for Hospice and
    Specialist Palliative Care Services
    120, 178, 180, 199
Neale, B. 9, 18, 122
Nuland, S. 182

O'Brien, T. 13
Oltjenburns, K. 13
Orona, C. 115, 116
Ortner, S. 58–9
Owens, P. 12

Parker, G. 122
Parry, J. 173–4
Pasteur, L. 141
Payne, S. 118, 119, 146, 200
Penso, D. 34
Pernick, R. 192
Pines, D. 131–2
Price, B. 115
Proctor, R. 202

Randall, F. 30
Ranger, T. 11
Reynolds Whyte, S. 195
Richardson, R. 9
Robillard, A. 164

Robinson, J. 194
Roper, M. 74
Rose, N. 5, 6, 13, 161
Rothfield, P. 203
Rowles, G. 99

Sabean, D. 63
Sacks, O. 197
Said, E. 111
Sartre, J. 87
Saunders, C.: (1965) 12, 15; (1986) 13, 15; (1988) 14, 15; (1992) 180; (1993) 179; influence 12, 15, 178, 193; pledge 14
Scarry, E. 181, 203
Schutz, A. 53
Scott, J. 143, 144
Seale, C.: (1989) 15, 18, 133; (1990) 9–10; (1998) 93, 132, 149, 178, 180, 182; and Addington-Hall (1995) 179
Seymour, J. 18, 180
Seymour, W. 87, 112, 162–4, 202
Shannon, T. 172
Sharma, U. 14
Sharpe, P. 83
Shaw, C. 194
Shilling, C.: (1991) 58, 196; (1993) 1, 7, 82, 83, 84, 175; and Mellor (1996) 102, 162
Shore, B. 5
Skeggs, B. 162
Skinner Cook, A. 13
Smaje, C. 34
Smith, A. 15, 115
Sontag, S. 168, 197
Standing Medical Advisory Committee and Standing Nursing and Midwifery Advisory Committee 144
Stein, A. 200
Stone, S. 110, 112
Strathern, M.: (1987) 101–2; (1988) 4, 109–10, 139–40; (1992a) 6, 192, 197; (1992b) 6, 60, 160, 197, 201
Strauss, A. 10, 15, 113, 119, 120, 153
Strong, P. 194
Sudnow, D. 10–11, 133, 153

Süskind, P. 136
Swedland, A. 196

Taylor, C. 5, 6
Taylor, C.C. 137, 140
Taylor, H. 17, 18–19, 23, 123, 199
Thomas, C. 61
Thomas Couser, G. 86, 183, 197
Thorpe, G. 122
Toombs, S. 47, 87, 89–90
Torrens, P. 19
Townsend, J. 122
Treichler, P. 14
Trezise, R. 47
Turner, B. 1, 82, 102, 162, 203
Turner, V. 82, 174
Twycross, R. 11, 12, 14–15

Ungerson, C. 61
Urla, J. 196

Van Gennep, A. 133, 174
Vialles, N. 144

Walker Bynum, C. 203
Walter, J. 172
Walter, T.: (1993) 11, 12; (1994) 9, 12–13, 14, 16, 18, 19, 132, 172
Watson, J. 174–5
Webb, C. 74
Weeks, J. 168
Weisman, A. 134, 171, 175
West, C. 167, 201
White, G. 61
White, P. 115
Wilkes, E. 19
Williams, S. 84, 162, 170, 196
Woodburn, J. 173
Woodhall, C. 128
Wright, S. 57–8

Younger, S. 115

Zaner, R. 115, 191
Zaretsky, E. 161
Zimmerman, D. 167, 201
Zola, I. 197
Zussman, R. 156

SUBJECT INDEX

abattoir 144
agency 101–3
alternative reality 41, 53, 57–61, 69, 71
Alzheimer's disease 115–16, 133
apathy 90, 93
autonomy: bodily 184; concept 165; loss of 37, 87, 124, 179; mutual 165

bed cutbacks 21, 22, 29, 80, 122–3
body: after death 21, 69–70, 174–5; boundaries 37, 87, 110–11, 128, 133, 137, 184; centrality 2–3; deterioration 66–7, 76, 87–9; in embodiment 82–7; fluids 140; illness and death 81; individuated 5; 'inscribed' 101; 'lived' 87, 101; loss of autonomy 37, 87, 124; mind–body dualism 2–3, 13, 81, 102; objectified bodies 105–12; performance 83, 163, 165; self and 36; transition to body-object 101–5; unbounded 128–9, 136, 141, 142–3; 'Western' 83–4, 104, 138–9
body-building 139
burden, being a 95–6

cancer patients 33, 119, 123, 133–4
Cancer Relief Macmillan Fund 75
care: concepts of 61–6, 72–5; packages 73
carers: interaction with high-dependency patients 184; obligation 165; perspectives and experiences 52, 105–12; sense of self 36
class: middle-class patients 22, 35, 168–9; paradox 168–70; working class patients 34–5, 169
comatose patients 113–14
communal group 55–6, 57, 59–60
conspiracy of silence 47
consumption behaviour 92
cosmetic surgery 45

day care: alternative reality 41, 53, 57–61, 69, 71; characteristics of patients 41–53; deterioration of patients 183; fieldwork 3–4, 25–9, 33; funding 23, 73–5, 80; goals 24, 25, 40; history 23; hospice movement 18; model of care 40, 57; re-referring patients 73; routine 55–7; safe retreat 35–6, 39, 40–1, 71; setting 54–5; space for masking deterioration and dependency 66–7, 76; space for sustaining the self 53–7
death: 'denial' of 69–72; dignified 179, 181; and dying in twentieth century 8–11; image of 16; impact on fellow patients 145–7; informing the patient 10, 11, 177; open confrontation 15–16, 117–19, 146–7; cross cultural perspectives 173–4; place of 78–9; social 38, 132, 148–9, 153–5, 178; taboo nature 123; talking about 34; as terminus 173; Western understanding of 173

dementia *see* Alzheimer's disease
dependency: masking 66–7;
    physical 51–3; relationships 65–6
dirt 136, 141
dress codes 60
dying: awareness off 34; bodily
    realities 37; definitions 113; fear
    of 171; 'living until you die' 14,
    37, 93, 116–17, 178; patient
    112–21; as a phase of liminality
    171–6; prolonged 172; public
    117–18; role 93; too soon 156–60;
    transition from subject to object
    87–96

embodiment *see* body
emotions 63–4
emotional labour *see* care
ethnic differences 34
euthanasia 113, 131, 132, 149,
    179–80

families: responses to deterioration
    and death 144–5; temporal
    frameworks 49–51
'family' metaphor 64–5
food and drink: commensality
    59–60; refusal of 130, 149, 152
Friends group 20
future, concept of 66, 67–9, 100

gender 35, 142–3, 149, 166–8

habitus 137, 169–70
Health Commission 73–5, 80, 122
high-dependency patients 93, 99,
    103, 105, 165, 184
Holocaust 131–2, 155–6
home care 18, 123
hospice: bed cutbacks 21, 22, 29,
    80, 122–3; deterioration of
    patients 183; development of
    movement 3–4, 11–16; discharges
    123; expansion and
    transformation 17–20; fieldwork
    3–4, 20–2, 29–33, 122; funding
    17–18, 80; goals 14, 116–17;
    movement 8; a 'no place' 143–5;
    taboos 143; working practices 80
house-bound patients 42–3

identity: loss of aspects of 2; person
    and self 4–8; self and 5
incontinence 129, 130–1, 135, 142
individual 4–6, 141, 173–4, 184
individualism 6–7, 83, 109, 138,
    141, 173
isolation: social 42, 43, 148, 164;
    temporal 46–51

liminality 133, 171–6
living too long 149–56, 179

Melanesian societies 109–10, 139
metaphors 64–5, 93–4, 128
mind–body dualism 2–3, 13, 81,
    102, 199
mobility 3, 87, 94–5, 164

National Health Service (NHS):
    funding strategies 3, 18; hospice
    provision 17–20
National Society for Cancer Relief
    (NSCR) 17–18, 20

odour *see* smells

pain: control 13, 22; total 13;
    unsharability 181–2
palliative care 18, 143–4, 176–82
past: references to 99–100;
    reminiscences of 68–9
persistent vegetative states (PVS)
    115
person: concept 2; individual and
    4–5; loss of 112–16, 142–3; self
    and identity 5–6; status 2; whole
    13
personal possessions 91–3
prosthetic devices 111–12, 184

quality of life 172

rehabilitation 24, 53
relationships: hierarchical 61–2;
    interpersonal 38, 148–9, 164–5
religious belief 34, 175–6
respite care 22, 123

St Christopher's hospice 12, 128
sedation 10–11, 119–21, 132, 149–50

self: concept 2, 15; disintegration of 32, 41–53, 166–70; identity and 5; loss of 89–90; making and unmaking through social connections 160–5; odyssey of 46; performance of 53, 83; person and identity 4–8; social relationships 38; space for sustaining 53–7; Western *see* Western
self-containment 3, 7, 136, 139
sexuality 168
single/side rooms 21–2, 29, 78–9, 119, 126, 147, 168–9
smells 22, 77, 126–8, 135–7, 164
spaces, shrinking 97–9
special case patients 157, 159
Steering Group 25
stigmatisation 44–5, 148, 163
suffering 172, 178, 181
switching off 131, 132

symptom control 22, 128–9

taboo(s): bodily 138, 144; death as 123; hospices 143
terminal: care 22; illness 47
therapeutic activities 24, 29, 56, 67
time: perceptions of 46–51, 67–8; shifts in perspectives 96–7; static 99–101

VE Day anniversary 99–100
volunteers 20, 25, 55–6, 189–90

wards: deaths in 79, 146–7; open 21, 29–30
'Western': body 83–4, 104, 138–9; healthcare provision 172; personhood 109, 110, 137, 138; self 1, 2, 3, 6–7, 52, 185; understanding of death 173
withdrawal 90, 93